Raw Food
CLEANSE

D0011089

Raw Food
CLEANSE

Restore Health and Lose Weight by Eating Delicious,
All-Natural Foods—Instead of Starving Yourself

PENNI SHELTON

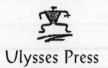

Ulysses Press

Text Copyright © 2010 Penni Shelton. Design Copyright © 2010 Ulysses Press and its licensors. All rights reserved under International and Pan-American Copyright Conventions, including the right to reproduce this book or portions thereof in any form whatsoever, except for use by a reviewer in connection with a review.

Published by: Ulysses Press
          P.O. Box 3440
          Berkeley, CA 94703
          www.ulyssespress.com

ISBN-13: 978-1-56975-742-0
Library of Congress Control Number: 2009930132

Printed in Canada by Transcontinental Printing

10 9 8 7 6 5 4 3 2 1

Acquisitions Editor: Keith Riegert
Managing Editor: Claire Chun
Editor: Hope Richardson
Editorial and production staff: Lauren Harrison, Judith Metzener
Cover design: what!design @ whatweb.com

Distributed by Publishers Group West

NOTE TO READERS
This book has been written and published strictly for informational purposes, and in no way should be used as a substitute for consultation with health-care professionals. You should not consider educational material herein to be the practice of medicine or to replace consultation with a physician or other medical practitioner. The author and publisher are providing you with information in this work so that you can have the knowledge and can choose, at your own risk, to act on that knowledge. The author and publisher also urge all readers to be aware of their health status and to consult health-care professionals before beginning any health program.

*To my precious family, for their unconditional love.
To God, for gifting me with the passion for natural healing
and the opportunity to share my heart with the world.
And to you, the reader. May you find something within
these pages of meaningful and lasting significance along
your journey for health and weight loss.*

Contents

Acknowledgments   ix

Foreword   xi

1   State of Our World   1

2   Our Human Condition:
The Cause & Effect of Our Toxic World   8

3   What We Should Be Eating Now   19

4   The Ultimate Raw Food Cleanse   33

5   Life Cleanse Recipes   46

6   Staying Detoxed in the Real World   141

7   Life Practices for Ageless Health   147

8   Real Stories from Raw Food Superheroes   166

Resources   225

References   231

Recipe Index   237

About the Author   244

Acknowledgments

This book is a culmination of the efforts and influence of many people who have educated, encouraged, led and loved me, and who have made the writing of this book possible. First, I would like to thank my friend Dhrumil Purohit—for without his help and belief in me, there would be no *Raw Food Cleanse*—and Ulysses Press, for taking a chance on me. I'd like to acknowledge my late mother-in-law, Virginia Shelton, as she was a true health pioneer and taught her boys the importance of choosing the best whole, fresh, local and organic foods available. I have certainly felt her guidance and presence as I've written this book.

I would like to thank Dr. Joel Robbins of Tulsa and Betsy Catrett of Daniel and Company for planting the good seeds that continue to produce a harvest in my life. Thanks to David Roth and Carol Alt for believing in me and putting my raw food journey "on the map." And to all my treasured friends across this globe who have encouraged and inspired me along the way, thank you.

A special thanks to Sunshine Boatwright for always being there, to Angela Thomas for being such a dear friend and my second pair of eyes, and to Susan Bradbury for her tireless support—and to all three for sharing and supporting my vision. A very special thank you to my beloved husband, Gordon, for allowing me the space in which to follow my heart's desire of teaching, traveling and writing, and to my father, Howard Collins, who has never stopped believing in me. And finally, to each cherished one who participated in the Raw Food Cleanse Experiment: the richness and depth of this body of work is because of you. Your stories will impact and change many lives. I love you all.

Foreword

The health of the world is suffering, there's no doubt about that. Degenerative diseases are on the rise, and for first the first time in human history, the current generation of youth will be less healthy than their parents' generation. Medical bills are the leading cause of bankruptcy, and if you watch the evening news, it can easily feel like things are quickly taking a turn for the worse.

Amongst all the fear, worry, and confusion though, there is a movement of people taking control of their own health and truly having fun doing it. This movement, however, wouldn't be possible without the wellness leaders who work so hard to research what works, to share their experiences, and to create practical programs for others to follow. I wholeheartedly consider Penni Shelton a driving force behind this movement and a premier example of a health educator who has no agenda other than to see people healthy and happy. She has the heart of a teacher and a personal testimony that millions can relate to.

Penni has written the *Raw Food Cleanse* to focus on the key to successful cleansing—quick gains and lots of momentum. Instead of a program that takes weeks for results to show, Penni's tiered cleansing protocol delivers results every step of the way. The 3-Day Energy Boost Cleanse will gently ease you into the world of cleansing and support you need so that you don't get overwhelmed by the detox process. Once you've had a taste of what true health feels likes, you'll be ready to take on a deeper cleanse that will deliver even more profound results. All along the way you'll be supported by the fantastic recipes in the book, which are so satisfying that you might actually forget you are cleansing. Most importantly, with each cleanse you do, you'll slowly begin to drop bad health habits that you never imagined you'd be able to leave behind—not because you have to, but because you'll want to. This is the power of cleansing. With every cleanse you take on, you teach your body to crave what is naturally best for it and in turn improve your overall health.

This book, and the cleanses featured in it, will not only help you lose weight and transform your relationship with food, but it will also radically change your definition of what it means to be truly healthy. I commend you for taking control of your wellness journey, and I wish you the best of success on your Raw Food Cleanse.

Dhrumil Purohit
We Like It Raw

1

State of Our World

Raw Food Cleanse is filled with nuggets of information and truth to help empower and educate you on how to achieve your own personal best, both in weight loss and in regaining your health. There is no magic bullet—just practical information on how to begin what has already been for many a life-changing journey to optimal health and permanent weight loss.

As we begin, it's important to take a realistic look at the standard American lifestyle and our environment, exploring how the two affect our overall health, well-being, and even our weight. It's also beneficial to gain perspective on the medical community and their role in your health and healing. In today's world, modern health-care professionals are able to keep us alive longer than they did 100 years ago, yet statistics show that the average American will live with a chronic degenerative disease for 20 years.

Catastrophic disease in America is epidemic. This year 35 percent of all deaths will be due to cardiovascular disease. At least one in four deaths are from cancer. Every single day, just under 8,000 people die from disease, which adds up to more American deaths annually than occurred during the entire Vietnam War. Over 4 million women are considered to be infertile. Depression, ADD, chronic fatigue syndrome, PMS and fibromyalgia affect 70 percent of American women over the age of 17.

Now let's consider obesity. The American Heart Association reports that among Americans 20 years old and older, 145 million Americans are overweight or obese. Over one third of American children are suffering from weight-related issues. The reality is that being overweight contributes to over 60 diseases.

Finally, an alarming statistic is that a significant cause of death in America is from adverse reactions to medications that were properly prescribed and taken correctly. The *New England Journal of Medicine* says that 2 million Americans fall ill and are hospitalized every year from reactions to prescription drugs. Of those 2 million, more than 140,000 die from that reaction. That puts adverse reactions in the same category as heart disease, cancer, diabetes and strokes as a top cause of premature death in America today.

It's not surprising that people are becoming more attuned to their own bodies and beginning to seek answers outside the sphere of modern medicine. Current statistics show that more and more Americans each year are seeking "alternative" medical approaches. Many individuals I meet are interested in finding ways to build their health and pinpoint the source of their illness. People have grown weary of repeated visits to the doctor just to manage symptoms.

All of that being said, as I travel and give lectures I'm careful not to be too critical of physicians and hospitals. If I were in a life-threatening accident, I would want to be rushed to the closest emergency facility, and I'd be very thankful to have a skilled physician, surgeon and nursing staff to care for me. Today's doctors are not evil, nor are their contributions trivial, as some natural health educators like to imply. Today's physicians have simply been taught, as we all have, that illness is normal and natural, especially as we age. Doctors fully expect that most people are simply going to get sick sooner or later.

The problem I see is not with the skilled health care workers themselves, but with the fact that they don't receive a thorough background in nutrition. Because of this, they place minimal value on the importance of food and the role it plays in health and healing. Doctors today are exhaustively trained in treating the symptoms of disease with pharmaceuticals, removing growths or cancers with surgical procedures and managing pain. However, there is not nearly enough emphasis on the statement made by the father of modern medicine, Hippocrates: "Let thy food be thy medicine and thy medicine be thy food."

My 16-year-old daughter was diagnosed with mild to moderate depression around the time she reached puberty. Her father and I made an appointment with a highly respected adolescent psychologist to discuss treatment options. Being the natural health advocate that I am, I broached the subject of diet and shared my concern regarding my teenager's poor food choices. I added that I thought there was a vitamin/mineral deficiency at play as well as social and situational concerns contributing to the problem. This professional and two other doctors we saw were not interested in discussing dietary changes or adding supplements to the list of possible treatments. They all felt that my daughter was a typical teenager, enjoying a diet rich in fast food, and that her daily choices of pizza, French fries, chocolate ice cream and soda had no bearing on her mental health.

It was through that trying experience, and others like it, that I learned the importance of knowing when to look to allopathic medicine and when to explore holistic treatments. Both can be viable options. Learning how to take charge of your own personal health and well-being, and that of your loved ones, is just another facet of achieving optimum health. I'm also encouraged as I learn of more cutting-edge, trailblazing physicians who are educating themselves and in turn offering their patients new options of care that combine holistic and Western medical traditions. I'm hopeful that we'll see this trend grow over time.

Exploring our society's dietary history helps enlighten us as to why we are faced with many of today's degenerative diseases. Before the 1940s, only a small percentage of the foods we ate were processed. Since 1940, the consumption of whole grains has decreased by at least 50 percent. The regular consumption of locally grown fresh fruits and vegetables has decreased by a startling amount, yet the quantity of sugar in our diet has doubled. The regular intake of processed foods has increased fourfold, and food-coloring additives are loaded into nearly everything packaged or processed. Soft drink consumption is up 300 percent since the 1940s, and currently 90 percent of the standard American diet is made up of foods that have been processed in some way. Statistics show that 90 percent of every food dollar is spent on processed foods. *Yikes*.

So, our body chemistry has evolved over millions of years, but our current lifestyle has only developed over the last hundred years, becoming even more dramatically altered after the Second World War. As our lives have become more modernized and hectic to meet the demands of this present age, our diets have followed suit. We began consuming an increased number of toxins and denatured foods, and our stress levels skyrocketed. In some very fundamental ways, modern civilization, with its mind-boggling technological advances, has actually compromised us more than it has helped us. Now we live in a society that eagerly accepts fast foods, even those that are heavily processed and loaded with chemicals, as a way of life for the average American, at any age.

Few people give any real thought to what they are actually eating as they cruise to the nearest drive-thru to get their daily fix of overly processed, denatured food that is devoid of most essential nutrients. The typical modern diet is proving to be more and more detrimental to our health. And the fact that many of our modern health-care professionals close their eyes to this reality in treating our illnesses, whether acute or degenerative, is cause for alarm. As a country we are getting sicker and sicker, even though we have the most advanced medical technology in the world. As we've already discussed, medical technology is geared toward treating symptoms, not identifying their causes.

I am still baffled that our universities and medical schools are not offering or requiring more nutritional curriculum. Research consistently shows that 85 percent of the degenerative diseases in this country are linked to poor lifestyle, in particular, to our diet. The vast majority of people would prefer to spend their money and energy looking for quick fixes rather than actually changing their lifestyle. I've heard it said that it's easier for a person to consider changing their religion than it is for them to make lasting changes to their diet. And a question I get asked all the time by skeptical friends and acquaintances is, "Does food *really* matter?" I believe it does.

There are natural laws and a natural order to this life. Our Creator designed it that way. Gravity is a perfect example. You may totally believe that you can leap from the top of a four-story building and fly; you may even be able to convince others of this. The reality is that if you do jump, you will hit the ground. Real health functions under the same kind of law. You may choose to eat a diet rich in animal fats, processed grains and sugars, caffeinated beverages and sports drinks, and even if you believe that it won't affect your health, eventually it will catch up to you.

Along with an evaluation of our diet, we must also examine the environmental dangers in today's world. The modernization of our society has not only created a massive amount of accommodating fast foods, it has also created other modern conveniences that have taxed our environment. There are many chemicals and other toxic materials that have been created largely by industry. These chemicals have infiltrated our water, our food and our precious air supply. Unfortunately we can't see, feel or smell many of these toxins. In many cases, people don't comprehend the effects these toxins have on our bodies until they receive a diagnosis of a chronic disease years after exposure.

The most encouraging news on the subject of environmental toxins is that there is a growing movement at a grassroots level that is bringing much of what is going wrong to the surface. Environmental activists and organizations are springing up all over the planet and the once faint voice is growing louder and stronger. More and more people are becoming aware of what is happening across our globe and how it is adversely affecting our health and the health of our young children. Although I see encouraging changes, more large-scale efforts are needed. I believe things will continue to evolve as we educate and empower ourselves and others.

It's true that industrialization within our culture has created poor dietary habits and a sick environment, but it has also brought with it another insidious factor that threatens our health. I am convinced that lifestyle stresses may be equally damaging, if not more so, to our overall health. The pressures of our everyday lives are at crisis levels, yet we have become so desensitized that the hectic way we live seems normal.

The overstimulation and the busy pace of a modern culture leads to emotional and relational imbalances, lack of exercise and poor elimination. A high percentage of people struggle with addictions of all kinds in an effort to just get through the day and cope. Although it is a sad state of affairs, it is within our grasp to transform and alter the course of our lives. We just have to recognize the need, then learn how to change and become empowered to do so. Knowledge is power, and my hope is that this little book will surprise you, give you hope, encourage and equip you with the practical tools to redirect your life onto the path of reclaiming your own optimal health. Many others have taken the step before you and I can't wait to share those stories with you as we go.

2

Our Human Condition: The Cause & Effect of Our Toxic World

As I talk with people from around the globe, I find awareness is growing as individuals realize that their mainstream diet, stressful lifestyle, and sick environment are contributing to an out-of-balance, compromised body. Although there is increased understanding in the health-conscious circles in which I speak and teach, it's clear that many people in the mainstream have yet to make the cause-and-effect connection between these damaging daily exposures and their ill health.

The purpose of this book is not to be negative or fatalistic; however, I believe it is of urgent importance to present the truth as clearly and accurately as possible based on current facts and research. In this chapter, we'll look at the main sources of toxins in your life and help you identify what steps are most crucial for you to take now in order to move toward your personal optimal health. Accurate information equips and inspires, and it is my hope that the truths presented here will be a catalyst for positive change and renewed health along your journey.

Did you know that over 77,000 chemicals are produced in North America? There are over 3,000 chemicals added to our food supplies, over 10,000 chemical solvents, emulsifiers and preservatives used for food processing, and over 1,000 new chemicals introduced each year. I don't know about you, but to me these numbers are pretty overwhelming.

So what effects do these toxins have on our bodies? A study by the British Medical Journal says that 75 percent of most cancers are caused by environmental and lifestyle factors. A report by the Columbia University School of Public Health estimates that 95 percent of cancer is caused by diet and environmental toxicity. I've read in numerous places that Americans have between 400 and 800 chemicals stored in their bodies, mainly in their fatty tissues. What are the short- and long-term effects of these toxins? Check this list out:

- Neurological disorders (Parkinson's, Alzheimer's, depression, ADD and ADHD, schizophrenia, etc.)
- Enzyme dysfunction
- Nutritional deficiencies
- Altered metabolism
- Hormonal imbalances
- Reproductive disorders
- Chronic fatigue
- Headaches/migraines
- Obesity
- Muscle and vision problems

- Suppressed immunity
- Allergies/asthma
- Endocrine disorders
- Chronic viral infections

Like me, you may be wondering what everyday chemicals are especially heinous to humans. Here is a list of the top 10 most common toxins found in our environment:

ASBESTOS   This insulating material was widely used from the 1950s to the 1970s. Problems arise when the material becomes old and crumbly and releases fibers into the air. Risks include scarring of the lung tissue and cancer, including a rare form of cancer called mesothelioma. Main sources of asbestos include insulation on floors and ceilings, water pipes and leaking ducts (especially in buildings from the 1950s–1970s).

CHLORINE   This highly toxic yellow-green gas is one of the most heavily used chemical agents. Risks include eye and skin irritation, severe eye and skin burns, blue coloring of the skin, sore throat, coughing, rapid breathing, narrowing of the bronchi, wheezing, accumulation of fluid in the lungs, pain in the lung region, lung collapse, and reactive airways dysfunction syndrome (RADS; a type of asthma). Main sources include household cleaners, public drinking water (even in small amounts), and air near factories that use chlorine in industrial processes (e.g., paper plants).

CHLOROFORM   This colorless liquid has a pleasant, nonirritating odor and a slightly sweet taste, and is used to make other chemicals. It's also formed when chlorine is added to water. Risks include cancer, reproductive damage, birth defects, dizziness, fatigue, headache, and liver and kidney damage. Air, drinking water, and food can contain chloroform.

DIOXINS These are chemical compounds formed as a result of combustion processes such as commercial or municipal waste incineration and from burning fuels (like wood, coal or oil). Risks include cancer, reproductive and developmental disorders, chloracne (a severe skin disease with acne-like lesions), skin rashes, skin discoloration, excessive body hair and mild liver damage. Over 95 percent of exposure comes from eating commercial animal fats.

HEAVY METALS Metals like arsenic, mercury, lead, aluminum and cadmium, which are prevalent in many areas of our environment, can accumulate in soft tissues of the body. Risks include cancer, neurological disorders, Alzheimer's disease, foggy head, fatigue, nausea and vomiting, decreased production of red and white blood cells, abnormal heart rhythm and damage to blood vessels. Main sources include public drinking water, fish, vaccines, pesticides, preserved wood, antiperspirant, building materials, dental amalgams and chlorine plants.

MOLD AND OTHER FUNGAL TOXINS Thirty-three percent of people have had an allergic reaction to mold. Mycotoxins (fungal toxins) can cause a range of health problems even with only a small exposure. Risks include cancer, heart disease, asthma, multiple sclerosis and diabetes. Main sources include contaminated buildings, foods like peanuts, wheat and corn, and alcoholic beverages.

PCBS (POLYCHLORINATED BIPHENYLS) This industrial chemical has been banned in the United States for decades, yet is an unrelenting organic pollutant that's still present in our environment. Risks include cancer and impaired fetal brain development. Avoid eating farm-raised salmon; they are fed meals of ground-up fish that have absorbed PCBs in the environment.

PESTICIDES   According to the Environmental Protection Agency (EPA), 60 percent of herbicides, 90 percent of fungicides and 30 percent of insecticides are known to be carcinogenic. I find it alarming that pesticide residues have been detected in 50 to 95 percent of U.S. foods. Risks include cancer, Parkinson's disease, miscarriage, nerve damage, birth defects, and blocked absorption of food nutrients. Main sources include bug sprays, conventional fruits and vegetables, and commercially raised meats.

PHTHALATES   These chemicals are used to lengthen the life of fragrances and soften plastics. Risks include endocrine system damage (phthalates chemically mimic hormones and are particularly dangerous to children). Plastic wrap, plastic bottles and plastic food-storage containers can leach phthalates into our food.

VOCS (VOLATILE ORGANIC COMPOUNDS)   VOCs are a major contributing factor to ozone, an air pollutant. According to the EPA, VOCs tend to be 200–500 percent more concentrated in indoor air than outdoor air, likely because they are present in so many household products. Risks include cancer, eye and respiratory tract irritation, headaches, dizziness, visual disorders and memory impairment. Main sources include drinking water, carpet, paints, deodorants, cleaning fluids, varnishes, cosmetics, dry-cleaned clothing, moth repellents and air fresheners.

I realize that this is a threatening list of dangerous pollutants; however, you can minimize your exposure and even overcome many of the injurious side effects by making mindful dietary and lifestyle changes. Although it's impossible to avoid all environmental toxins, you can drastically limit your exposure to them. The information in

Chapter 6 will help you formulate a game plan for reducing your exposure and taking your detox to a deeper level.

To determine your personal toxic load, start by answering the following questions, which were designed to help you understand what offenders may be contributing to your weight or health challenges.

Text continued on page 19.

LIFE CLEANSE QUESTIONNAIRE
DIETARY PROFILE

Do you regularly consume …	DAILY	OCCASIONALLY (less than 3x/wk.)	RARELY	NEVER
Commercial, Pasteurized dairy products (milk, cheese, butter, eggs, ice cream, etc.):				
As a child/adult	☐	☐	☐	☐
In the last 2 years	☐	☐	☐	☐
Commercially raised meats (beef, pork, chicken, fish, turkey, etc.):				
As a child/adult	☐	☐	☐	☐
In the last 2 years	☐	☐	☐	☐
Processed enriched grains (cereal, bagels, pastries, crackers, waffles, pancakes, etc.):				
As a child/adult	☐	☐	☐	☐
In the last 2 years	☐	☐	☐	☐
Processed, refined sugar (white sugar, high-fructose corn syrup, etc.):				
As a child/adult	☐	☐	☐	☐
In the last 2 years	☐	☐	☐	☐
Non-organic soy products (tofu, soy milk, soy meats, non-organic edamame, etc.):				
As a child/adult	☐	☐	☐	☐
In the last 2 years	☐	☐	☐	☐
"Fake foods" (anything containing food coloring, artificial sweeteners, chemicals. Products like; Twinkies, Spam, Velveeta, powdered drink mixes, candy, and other highly processed items):				
As a child/adult	☐	☐	☐	☐
In the last 2 years	☐	☐	☐	☐
Coffee, black tea, soft drinks, sports drinks and/or bottled juices:				
As a child/adult	☐	☐	☐	☐
In the last 2 years	☐	☐	☐	☐

The longer and more often you have consumed the above, the greater your toxic load and the higher your chances of being overweight and in compromised health.

PHYSICAL HEALTH

Do you consider yourself a yo-yo dieter or has your weight fluctuated more than 10% in either direction repeatedly in your adult life?	☐ YES	☑ NO
Are you over 40 years of age?	☑ YES	☐ NO
Do you consider yourself "regular"? (1 or more bowel movements daily)	☑ YES	☐ NO

Do you currently have any of the following health conditions?

Overweight—25 pounds or more:	☐ YES	☑ NO
Overweight—75 pounds or more:	☐ YES	☑ NO
High cholesterol:	☐ YES	☑ NO
High blood pressure:	☐ YES	☑ NO
Diabetes:	☐ YES	☑ NO
Asthma or other respiratory mucosal condition:	☐ YES	☑ NO
IBS or other bowel disorder:	☐ YES	☑ NO
Heartburn or other digestive condition:	☐ YES	☑ NO
Insomnia:	☐ YES	☑ NO
Migraines:	☐ YES	☑ NO
Osteoporosis:	☐ YES	☑ NO
Arthritis:	☑ YES	☐ NO
Depression:	☐ YES	☑ NO
Chronic pain:	☐ YES	☑ NO
Ulcers:	☐ YES	☑ NO
Liver disease/cirrhosis:	☐ YES	☑ NO
Stroke:	☐ YES	☑ NO
Kidney disease:	☐ YES	☑ NO
Thyroid disease:	☐ YES	☑ NO
Heart disease:	☐ YES	☑ NO
Cancer:	☐ YES	☑ NO

Fluctuating weight, irregularity, being moderately overweight to severely obese and living with a body that is taxed by any of the above health conditions are all symptoms that you are struggling with a toxic load. The more the body ages, gains weight and retains toxicity, the more its systems begin to breakdown.

BODY MOVEMENT

Do you get 20 to 30-plus minutes of aerobic exercise 5 times a week? (walking, running, swimming, biking, rebounding, etc.) ☐ YES ☐ NO

Do you participate in 20-plus minutes of strength/resistance training at least 3 times a week? (weight-lifting, resistance bands, circuit equipment, etc.) ☐ YES ☐ NO

Do you participate in 30-plus minutes of flexibility movement 3 times a week? (yoga, Pilates, stretching, etc.) ☐ YES ☐ NO

Lack of body movement adds to the sluggishness of one's internal systems and creates a deficit in essential oxygen entering the bloodstream.

ENVIRONMENTAL CONDITIONS

Do you now or have you ever worked in an environment in which you are regularly exposed to chemicals or solvents? ☐ YES ☐ NO

Do you use or carry a mobile phone on your body for 1 or more hours daily? ☐ YES ☐ NO

Do you work on a computer or sit close to a computer for more than 2 hours daily? ☐ YES ☐ NO

Do you have regular (1 to 2 times a year) x-rays, mammograms, MRIs, or other such contact with radiation/x-rays? ☐ YES ☐ NO

Do you live in or near a large city? ☐ YES ☐ NO

Many experts agree that electromagnetic fields (EMFs) are a threat to our health. Even the Environmental Protection Agency (EPA) warns "There is reason for concern" and advises "prudent avoidance."

SPIRITUAL LIFE

Do you regularly attend a church, synagogue, temple, mosque or other place of worship? ☐ YES ☐ NO

Do you engage in regular prayer, meditation or other such spiritual practice? ☐ YES ☐ NO

Do you take time to rest and reflect on your personal blessings or use positive affirmations? ☐ YES ☐ NO

Do you feel a connection or have an awareness of God, the Creator or a higher power on a daily basis? ☐ YES ☐ NO

Dan Buettner, author of The Blue Zones: Lessons for Living Longer from the People Who've Lived the Longest, *cites one of the secrets to longevity and health as living a life which incorporates spiritual purpose, religion and a community of faith.*

EMOTIONAL FACTORS

Within the last 12 months have you had any of the following occur:

Serious illness: ☐ YES ☐ NO

Close family member with a serious illness: ☐ YES ☐ NO

Recently lost a close loved one to death: ☐ YES ☐ NO

Separation/divorce: ☐ YES ☐ NO

Serious legal trouble: ☐ YES ☐ NO

Career change: ☐ YES ☐ NO

Moved primary residence: ☐ YES ☐ NO

New baby or other person(s) joined your household: ☐ YES ☐ NO

Serious family/relationship problems: ☐ YES ☐ NO

Serious financial stress: ☐ YES ☐ NO

Served as primary caregiver of someone ill/disabled ☐ YES ☐ NO

Are you happy in your primary relationship?
(Marriage/cohabitation) ☐ YES ☐ SOMEWHAT ☐ NO

Do you have a satisfying level
of intimacy in your life? ☐ YES ☐ SOMEWHAT ☐ NO

Are you satisfied in your current field of daily work?
(Career, homemaker, student, etc.) ☐ YES ☐ SOMEWHAT ☐ NO

Do you have close, meaningful, harmonious
friendships? ☐ YES ☐ SOMEWHAT ☐ NO

Do you have pets? ☐ YES ☐ NO

Are you involved in a community in which you serve, build
relationships or gain support?
(PTA, charity, social or recreational group, etc.) ☐ YES ☐ NO

Life stress and troubled or inadequate relationships can deeply affect our state of well-being and health. It's good to honestly evaluate what you can do to adjust and heal areas that may be out of balance.

LIFESTYLE

Do you now or have you ever had a dependency on drugs
or alcohol? ❑ YES ❑ NO

Have you taken birth control, antibiotics, pain medications,
anti-depressants or other prescription drugs for 3+ months
in your past? ❑ YES ❑ NO

Do you currently take any prescription drugs daily? ❑ YES ❑ NO

Do you currently smoke? ❑ YES ❑ NO

Are you around others who smoke daily? ❑ YES ❑ NO

Do you currently use recreational drugs? ❑ YES ❑ NO

Do you have more than 5 alcoholic beverages weekly? ❑ YES ❑ NO

Do you now or have you ever had an eating disorder? ❑ YES ❑ NO

Do you sleep less than 8 hours most nights? ❑ YES ❑ NO

Do you get less than 15 minutes of sunlight daily? ❑ YES ❑ NO

Do you drink less than half your body weight in ounces
of water (including herbal tea or fresh juice) daily? ❑ YES ❑ NO

*Research has shown that tobacco, alcohol or substance abuse, as well
as eating disorders, are linked to long-range poor overall health. Lack
of adequate sleep and sunlight, along with chronic dehydration, also
produce an atmosphere in which the body cannot regain a state of
equilibrium to begin the healing process.*

3

What We Should Be Eating Now

You are what you eat, right? Well, the real truth is that we are what we eat, digest and assimilate. Learning to enjoy foods in their natural, fresh, raw state is the best way to ensure that you will digest and assimilate the most nutrients possible. The processing of food strips it of its essential nutrients by overheating and oxidation—and then there's the addition of toxic materials. Nature designed our foods in a complete package with all the nutrients and enzymes needed to digest and assimilate them into a usable state. When whole foods are stripped of part of the original package, they become nutrient-draining to our bodies rather than life-giving and nutrient-dense. Unfortunately, our bodies must be robbed of needed nutrients and enzymes in order to break down this denatured food.

Choosing mostly fresh, raw, organic and locally harvested foods, like those you'd find at a farmers' market, makes for an ideal diet. If there are no farmers' markets near you selling locally grown, seasonal fruits and vegetables, the next best choice is to support grocers like Whole Foods or other healthy natural food stores. Conventionally grown produce is often deficient in nutrients for a number of reasons. The soil is often overworked and lacking in minerals; the vegetation has generally been treated with multiple pesticides, herbicides, larvicides, fungicides and chemical fertilizers; and produce has often been shipped from around the world.

Aside from eating fresh, raw whole foods, the next best way to maximize nutrition for your body is through juicing or blending whole foods. The freshly extracted juices of fruits and vegetables deliver easily assimilated, instant nutrients into the system. No matter how challenged one's digestion may be, juicing is the definitive way to maximize the absorption of vitamins, minerals and amino acids. Even the most compromised, sickly, nutrient-deficient body can greatly benefit from juiced and blended raw whole foods. Acclaimed health retreats around the world utilize juicing in the healing and detoxification process of their patients. There are volumes of documented cases of cancers and other degenerative diseases being successfully treated and healed with the nutritional support of fresh vegetable and fruit juices.

One must consume fresh juices immediately after extracting. Once the skin of a fruit or vegetable is broken, oxidation begins and the food begins to lose nutritional value. We desperately need these live and active enzymes in order to help rejuvenate and repair our bodies. Although often underrated by doctors and nutritionists, enzymes are vital players in helping you regain your most vibrant health.

Along with juicing, drying or dehydrating is another nutrient-maximizing food preparation. Drying has been used as a method of preserving foods for thousands of years and by many cultures. Long before the invention of refrigeration, people were putting fresh foods into the sun to dry so they could enjoy them at a later time. Dehydrated foods keep and travel well, but look for foods that have been dried with no chemicals or additives. Foods that have been dried at less than 115 degrees retain about 95 percent or more of their nutritional value, which makes them a great staple to store for the winter. A dehydrator is a money-saving purchase if you're committed to improving the integrity of your health (see the Resources section for more information).

What about eating frozen foods? Obviously it's not always possible to find fresh produce, especially in the winter months, so freezing or buying frozen is a suitable option. Do you read labels when buying frozen produce? Choose organic whenever possible and look for companies that flash freeze immediately after picking. Frozen foods retain 70 to 95 percent of their nutrients, depending on the freezing practice.

Although this book is titled *Raw Food Cleanse*, lightly steamed foods can be a healthy alternative when you desire warm foods in the colder months. Be careful not to over-steam. When steamed foods begin to lose color and feel limp, they are overcooked and have lost a significant amount of their nutritional value.

Any preparation that heats food to over 115 degrees depletes all of the living enzymes that help your body digest and assimilate what you swallow. Depending upon how long you cook your food, this process will not only kill all the living enzymes, it will also cause a 50 to 100 percent depletion of the nutrients in your food. I find that people are resistant if you tell them that baking, broiling, grilling or steaming foods for too long limits the body's ability to process them efficiently. But even my husband, a self-proclaimed grilling master, has started being more mindful of how long he leaves his food on the fire.

Microwaved leftovers, commercially canned foods and fried foods have all lost close to 100 percent of their nutritional value. Processed cooked foods with additives, which make up a huge portion of the typical American diet, not only have zero nutritional value, they also have toxins added to them that significantly increase your chances of degenerative illness. I am convinced that this is why we have a country filled with overfed, undernourished adults and children. People keep eating, plugging themselves until they're stuffed with nutrient-depleted foods, but they are still hungry. Their bodies are crying out for the vital nutrition that satisfies, nourishes and heals.

A big missing link in mainstream approaches to weight loss and health is the study of the acid/alkaline balance. It you've consumed a typical American diet for any significant length of time, you are most likely dealing with an acid issue. One of the main goals of the Raw Food Cleanse is to move your body out of its acidic state and into a more alkaline environment.

Are You Too Acidic?

The following foods and lifestyle choices may lead to an acid problem.

- Meat, including chicken, pork, turkey and fish
- Dairy products, including eggs
- Bread, pasta, potatoes, and baked goods
- Cigarettes and other forms of tobacco
- Alcohol, prescription and recreational drugs

- Coffee and most commercial teas
- Processed or fast foods
- Sugar
- Artificial sweeteners
- Soft drinks and sports drinks
- No exercise
- Stress, negative emotions and spiritual emptiness

Another factor that stalls weight loss is dehydration. High acid levels and lack of hydration have something in common. Check this out: Your body retains fat as a protection against the acids produced by the lifestyle outlined in the above list. Some of the acids are eliminated through the bowels, urinary tract and skin, but whatever is left behind has to be buffered and neutralized. In the same way your body manages to sustain an ideal body temperature of around 98.6 degrees, your body also intrinsically knows to maintain a pH balance that is within very precise boundaries. Your ingeniously created system goes to impressive lengths to keep you in balance by storing fat, building cholesterol plaque, draining calcium from bones, and leaching magnesium out of your heart or muscles. This all happens as your body battles to protect against acid damage.

The human body is composed of approximately 65 percent water, which means that we're made up of somewhere between 10 and 13 gallons of water. We've already said that we are what we eat, but we are also quite literally what we drink. When you're dehydrated, your body goes into preservation or fat-storing mode. Every day that you don't drink enough water or drink the wrong things, you put your body at additional risk and on some level compromise your health. If your body has been dealing with a major acid intake, your fat is actually protecting your cells, tissues and organs. This may be a new perspective, but there's a good chance that your stored fat is actually working to save your life!

In a nutshell, along with consuming an acid-forming diet, being dehydrated can likely lead to weight gain. There is also a tendency for the body to send confusing signals to your brain. An example of this is that many of us mistake thirst/dehydration for hunger, so we eat when we really need to be drinking. If we don't get enough water, our bodies actually retain water and feel bloated and uncomfortable. Lack of water is the number-one cause of daytime fatigue. Do you recognize any of these symptoms?

Symptoms of Dehydration

- Weakness and fatigue
- Problems focusing and concentrating
- Drowsiness
- Impatience and irritability
- Headaches or migraines
- Brain fog; clouded thinking
- Short-term memory loss
- Trouble articulating
- Lightheadedness
- Cold hands and feet
- Anxiety
- Depression

Besides the above list, degenerative conditions including morbid obesity, heart disease and cancer are all linked with serious long-term dehydration. Sounds shocking, but it's true.

So the question is, how much water should you be drinking? Half your body weight in ounces daily is optimal, which means that if you weigh 200 pounds you should be drinking 100 ounces of pure water each day. If you are very active or out in the hot sun for extended periods, this amount needs to increase. The good news is that you may also count any freshly extracted fruit and vegetable juices, herbal teas and the liquid from young coconuts toward your daily total.

I hope you have followed my train of thought regarding proper hydration and the importance of re-alkalinizing your body. Many studies and reports are being released showing that cancer and other degenerative diseases can't survive in an alkaline environment.

In order to cleanse the body and lose weight for good, we must transition away from the typical American diet. Setting a goal of eating 80 percent whole, fresh, raw, ripe, organic focus foods will give you amazing results. As we've seen, these foods are the healthiest for your body due to their nutritional profiles and their alkaline-forming properties. They are the healing and life-giving foods that your body needs to rejuvenate, restore health and bring your body into homeostasis.

The other 20 percent of your diet is up to your common sense. People with compromised immunity, those who are obese, individuals with degenerative disease, and those with severe food allergies or sensitivities will likely need to consider carefully how they approach this 20 percent. Many will choose to be 100 percent raw—and will generally reap faster results in doing so—while others prefer to use this 20 percent for social dining occasions, when traveling, and in other situations to help them function more comfortably in society.

Whatever you choose, it is important to let wisdom, not impulse, guide you in what you choose to put into your mouth. Your body is your temple. It is a gift and it's the only one you will get in this life. Stocking your refrigerator and pantry for success and being prepared daily is the key to your best diet. Be an example to others of what's possible. Be the influence; don't be the one who *is* influenced!

Here is the list of focus foods that are recommended while on any of the Raw Food Cleanse options. I encourage you to scan these pages and take them with you on trips to the grocery store.

Raw Food Cleanse Focus Foods

GREENS AND LEAFY GREENS

Arugula, asparagus, basil, broccoli, butter lettuce, cabbage, celery, cilantro, collard greens, cucumber, dandelion, lamb's quarters, leaf lettuce, leeks, kale, mint, parsley, peas, purslane, romaine, spinach, sprouts, watercress

VEGETABLES

Beets, bell peppers, carrots (organic only), cauliflower, celery, daikon, eggplant, garlic, ginger, jalapeño, onions, parsnips, radishes, scallions, shallots, squash, sweet potatoes, tomatillos, tomatoes, zucchini

FRUITS

Apples, apricots, bananas, berries (all kinds), cherries, goji berries, grapefruit, grapes, kiwis, lemons, limes, mangoes, melons (all kinds), oranges, papayas, peaches, pears, persimmons, pineapples

SEAWEEDS

Arame, dulse, hijiki, kelp, kombu, Irish moss, nori, wakame

GOOD FATS/OILS

Avocado, borage, coconut (young), cold-pressed extra virgin olive oil, evening primrose, flax, grapeseed, hemp, Udo's Choice

NUTS/SEEDS

Almond, cashew, chia, flax, hemp, macadamia, pumpkin, sesame

GRAINS/LEGUMES

Buckwheat, lentils, oats (preferably gluten-free), quinoa, wild rice

CONDIMENTS/SPICES

Apple cider vinegar, Celtic sea salt, cinnamon, lavender, miso, sauerkraut, umeboshi vinegar, vanilla

HERBAL TEAS

Chamomile, nettle, peppermint, rooibos, etc.

In the Resources section, you'll find a list of raw-food-friendly staples that are helpful to add to your pantry. It is in your long-range best interest to start crowding out the old processed foods with fresh, delicious, life-giving alternatives. I also recommend the following alkaline-forming superfoods that will support your immunity, fight disease and encourage lasting weight loss.

Alkaline-forming Superfoods

YOUNG THAI COCONUTS

One of the most powerful superfoods to help with both hydration and alkalinity is the young Thai coconut. The liquid within a young coconut is the most incredible, pure, delicious water. It is one of the richest sources of electrolytes known to man. Forget the commercial sports drinks! This amazing water, or milk, as some call it, is nearly identical to blood plasma. When we drink fresh coconut water, it's as if we've given ourselves an instant blood transfusion. Young coconuts are preferable to the more mature brown coconuts; they are most health-enhancing in their early stages of growth.

The meat of the young coconut contains lauric acid, known for its beneficial antimicrobial effects. Coconut meat and coconut oil do not contain trans-fatty acids. Most of the saturated fat in coconut oil consists of medium-chain fatty acids. This good fat gets digested and assimilated more easily: it is less likely to be stored in the body as fat and can actually help you burn more fat. In addition to antiviral and antibacterial properties, natural coconut fat helps normalize body lipids, protects against liver damage and, most importantly, improves the immune system's anti-inflammatory response. Good saturated fats such as these also contain micronutrients and vitamins that are vital to metabolism. Young coconuts can be found in most health food stores and Asian markets, or you can find organic sources online.

CHIA SEEDS

Nothing compares to the chia seed when it comes to hydration and endurance. Once soaked, these tiny seeds open up and absorb nine times their volume in water. The seeds, once fully hydrated, form a gel that is phenomenal at keeping your body hydrated. This gel is also 90 percent soluble fiber, which is beneficial for your digestive tract and helps to lower cholesterol even more effectively than oatmeal. And talk about an impressive nutritional profile:

the seeds have twice the protein of any other seed or grain, five times the calcium of milk, and copious amounts of omega-3 and omega-6, essential oils for the body. Because of the soluble fiber in the gel, incorporating chia into one's diet is very helpful for people with diabetes: the gel forms a wall around ingested carbohydrates, causing them to be released more gradually. Savvy dieters love the seeds because the gel can be added to foods or drinks without changing their flavor, and it helps provide a feeling of fullness and satisfaction. Using the hydrated seeds is an excellent way to control one's appetite. Although these seeds have superstar status, they are very affordable and are carried at most health food stores.

One word of warning: Don't use chia seeds unless you have soaked them for at least 10 minutes. If you eat them dry, they will actually use your bodily fluid to expand, and that can cause digestive issues and dehydration.

BEE POLLEN

Along with local raw honey, bee pollen is one of the most amazing foods you will ever eat. My friends Gabriel Cousens and David Rainoshek, both well-respected in the natural health movement, share the opinion that bee pollen contains all the elements necessary for the sustenance of human life. The San Francisco Medical Research Foundation estimates that pollen has more than 5,000 different enzymes and co-enzymes—more than any other food in existence.

The high amount of enzymes, such as catalase, amylase, and pectin-splitting enzymes, make pollen an aid to digestion. Some research suggests that pollen is absorbed directly from the stomach into the bloodstream. Pollen is a vegetarian source of human-active B12, most of the B vitamins, vitamins A, C, D and E, rutin, lecithin, all the essential amino acids, the essential fatty acid called linoleic acid, fats, complex carbohydrates, simple sugars, and many other beneficial agents that are still being studied.

According to research by doctors from France, Italy, and the former Soviet Union, pollen is the richest source of protein in nature. Gram for gram, pollen contains an estimated five to seven times more protein than meat, eggs or cheese. The protein in pollen is in a predigested form and therefore easy to assimilate.

When you try it for the first time, simply place a couple of granules under your tongue to check for any allergic response. (Only about 1 to 2 percent of the population is allergic to bee pollen.) You can find pollen at Whole Foods Market or online (see the Resources section for a list of recommended online retailers).

HEMP SEEDS

Hemp seeds contain all the essential amino and fatty acids necessary to maintain healthy human life. No other single plant source has the essential amino acids in such an easily digestible form, or the essential fatty acids in such a perfect ratio to meet human nutritional needs. As one of nature's most perfect foods, hemp seeds contain all 10 essential amino acids, the building blocks of protein. Hemp is also rich in naturally balanced omega-3 and omega-6 essential fatty acids, not to mention magnesium, iron, potassium, fiber and phytonutrients, plus natural antioxidants like vitamin E.

I highly recommend hemp seeds, as they are one of the plant kingdom's best sources of easily digestible, high-quality protein. To my knowledge, these amazing seeds are the highest vegan source of simple protein, which is required for proper immune system function.

Hemp is the perfect alternative protein, much less likely to cause allergic reactions and much less mucus-forming than dairy and soy sources. Adding hemp protein to your morning smoothie is a great way to support your entire system and power up for your day. Many vegan super-athletes supplement their daily dietary regime with hemp and spirulina.

SPIRULINA

Spirulina is both a food from the past and a food for the future. Some scientists speculate that the manna of the wandering Israelites, which appeared miraculously on rocks following a devastating dry spell and was described as tasting like wafers made with honey, may in fact have been a form of dried, dormant spirulina.

Spirulina is an exceptional food and an incredible source of concentrated, absorbable nutrients. Because it is 65 to 70 percent complete protein with all essential amino acids in perfect balance, it's a highly beneficial substitute for protein powders. This amazing blue-green algae also contains vitamins A, B1, B2, B6, B12, E and K. In addition, spirulina provides minerals, trace minerals, cell salts, phytonutrients and enzymes, as well as an abundance of chlorophyll and other beneficial pigments.

Beef is only 22 percent protein and is very difficult for most individuals to digest and assimilate. Even soybeans are only 34 percent protein. This makes spirulina one of the world's highest known sources of usable protein.

The reason I believe that vegan sources of protein are superior is that proteins from animals form relatively large amounts of uric acid, which can contribute to osteoporosis, gout, arthritis, lack of energy, acidic body chemistry, aging and more! Add powdered spirulina to your smoothies, juices, soups and sprinkle it on your salads for an intense source of nutrient density and added protein daily.

WHEATGRASS

Wheatgrass is an amazing blood purifier, cleanser and detoxifier. It contains chlorophyll, which helps carry oxygen to every cell in your body. Oxygen in the body's cells helps fight off harmful bacteria and diseases—even the most insidious diseases, like cancer. Wheatgrass must be squeezed, juiced or blended, and strained in order to assimilate its nutrients.

Wheatgrass is grown from the wheat seed or wheat berry, which is farmed in almost every U.S. state and around the globe. People with wheat allergies need not be concerned about consuming wheatgrass juice; it is a leafy green that is different from the grain and refined-grain products. This super-grass is also a complete protein with meganutrients when grown in an organic soil base.

My well-respected friends at the Hippocrates Health Institute suggest drinking wheatgrass juice in small amounts throughout the day, always on an empty stomach. Two to four ounces every day is sufficient. Slowly sipping small quantities of the juice will give your body an opportunity to get used to its taste and effects. Taking one to two ounces straight or mixed into other green juices or smoothies and sipping slowly will prevent nausea or upset stomach, as this is one of nature's most powerful detoxing and revitalizing agents. In addition to the Raw Food Cleanse dietary protocols, I suggest drinking one or two ounces of wheatgrass up to three or four times per day with one day of rest periodically. Although, be advised: with wheatgrass, more is not better. Two ounces at any one given time is all one person needs.

4

The Ultimate Raw Food Cleanse

This segment of the book is devoted to a number of different dietary cleanses. Depending on what you learned about yourself as you answered the Life Cleanse Questionnaire in Chapter 2, and based on your own personal needs for cleansing and weight loss, you can choose from among several options. Here you will find a **3-Day Energy Boost Cleanse**, **7-Day Rejuvenation Cleanse**, **14-Day Deep Detox Cleanse** and, finally, a **28-Day Total Body Reset Cleanse** for those with more serious detox issues and with the most weight to lose.

Regardless of where you are right now, I suggest you begin with the 3-Day Energy Boost Cleanse. If your body is taxed with a heavy toxic load and/or you have a substantial amount of weight to lose, you may experience some symptoms of detox as you begin cleansing. Starting with a three-day cleanse is a perfect way for you to learn how your body will react to this process of freeing up energy for detox. While some people experience headaches, nausea, body aches, digestive disturbances and other symptoms, others report absolutely no adverse reactions while cleansing. It is strictly up to you to decide the best way to approach the Raw Food Cleanse, either cautiously or by diving headfirst into the deep end of the raw-food pool!

One of my Raw Food Cleanse research participants, 45-year-old Dennis Clark, had absolutely no ill effects as he began cleansing. Dennis started the Raw Food Cleanse at just under 500 pounds and within 11 weeks he released 65 pounds. Needless to say, Dennis was so thrilled and motivated by his results, he has maintained a very high raw foods diet as a long-term lifestyle change. At the time of print, Dennis continues his impressive weight-loss journey and has become an emissary of the healthy transformations that are possible with a high-raw-foods diet.

All the recipes in these cleanses can be found in Chapter 5, Section I—The Raw Food Cleanse. And you can let your cleanse suit your tastes. Make any of the Raw Cleanse smoothies, juices or entrées you'd like, unless otherwise noted.

All cleanses should be combined with the lifestyle practices outlined in Chapter 7. Your ultimate success will be greatly enhanced as you practice daily body movement, pay attention to your daily elimination, care for your body and skin, receive adequate sunlight and create a daily space for prayer/meditation and for finding a sense of community.

3-Day Energy Boost

Day 1

It's generally best to start on a Friday, or when you are going to have a couple of days free from heavy daily demands.

Upon waking   Drink 32 ounces of pure, alkaline water with lemon to flush your system and help you wake up. You will continue to drink pure water throughout the day, keeping track and working toward your personal goal in ounces depending upon your body weight.

Breakfast   Have a Raw Cleanse smoothie or a bowl of fresh mixed fruit. Eat as much as desired.

Lunch   Have a Raw Cleanse salad. You may choose any dressing from the recipes section, or use a simple mixture of cold-pressed olive oil, lemon juice and Celtic sea salt.

After work/In the evening   Drink one or two cups of a mild laxative tea, like Smooth Move, with fresh lemon.

Dinner   Consume an all-raw dinner. Begin with fruits, preferably low-glycemic (berries, stone fruits), then prepare a large mixed-green salad with plenty of veggies (cucumber, bell pepper, tomato, avocado, sprouts, etc.). Again, make a dressing with olive oil, lemon juice and Celtic sea salt. Check out the recipes in Chapter 5, Section I—The Raw Food Cleanse for ideas.

Bedtime   Go to bed by 10 p.m. Your goal is eight hours of quality sleep.

Day 2

If you are able to schedule a deep-tissue massage or time in a sauna or steam room, this will be very beneficial. Doing an enema or having colon hydrotherapy would also enhance your experience and reduce any uncomfortable detoxing symptoms that could begin to manifest.

Upon waking Start off with 32 ounces of pure, clean water with lemon.

Breakfast Energize and detoxify with 16 ounces of alkalinizing green-based juice. See the list of juice recipes in Chapter 5, Section I—The Raw Food Cleanse.

Mid-morning Exercise if possible, either a brisk walk or 15 minutes on a mini-trampoline. When you're done, drink another 16 ounces of green juice.

Lunch Enjoy another Raw Cleanse salad, with the dressing of your choice.

After lunch, prepare Balancing Broth (page 76) for tonight's dinner.

Mid-afternoon Enjoy an herbal tea, a Smart Cocktail or an Ecstatic Elixir. Rest or nap for one hour if possible.

Dinner Have a large bowl of Balancing Broth (page 76) and another Raw Cleanse salad. Try to select a dressing that has avocado as the base for some needed essential fatty acid.

Bedtime In bed by 10 p.m.—going for eight hours of sleep!

Day 3

Upon waking Drink 32 ounces of pure water with lemon. Also plan to consume the correct amount of water throughout the day.

Breakfast Prepare a Green Smoothie (page 55) and drink 16–32 ounces of this throughout the morning.

Mid-morning   Try to get 30 minutes of exercise, and be sure to drink herbal tea and/or water to replenish afterward.

Lunch   Enjoy another bowl of last night's Balancing Broth (page 76) along with an Orange Spinach Salad with Orange Tahini Dressing (page 69).

Mid-afternoon   Have a Green Smoothie (page 55) and try to get in some rest time.

Dinner   Start with a Smart Cocktail or an Ecstatic Elixir, if desired. Then make a salad on a bed of mixed greens with grated carrot, beets and purple cabbage. Choose either a basic or avocado-based dressing. Have a side of steamed broccoli and onions with Bragg Liquid Aminos.

Bedtime   In bed by 10 p.m. Aim for eight hours of sleep!

7-Day Rejuvenation Cleanse

In my opinion, many people need more than just a 3-Day Energy Boost Cleanse. If you are recovering from a lifetime of poor diet and lifestyle choices, or detoxing from taxing environmental exposures, you should consider doing a 7-Day Rejuvenation Cleanse at least twice a year. This cleanse will give your vital body systems a chance to rest, restore and rejuvenate.

Aside from a good juicer and blender, all that is needed to successfully complete this seven-day cleanse is a bit of planning and the decision to make it happen. When undertaking any of the Raw Food Cleanses, most people appreciate the convenience of not having to take time off work or spend much money. All it takes is your commit-

ment to this cleanse that will help you rebalance, lose weight and achieve a newfound sense of well-being and mental clarity.

As with all of the cleanses outlined in this book, you should always begin your day with 32 ounces of pure, clean water and stay conscious of consuming adequate, quality fluids throughout each day. It is essential that you stay hydrated!

Daily Schedule

Intake before noon   Your choice of:

- 32-ounce Life Cleanse juice or
- 32-ounce Life Cleanse smoothie or
- 16-ounce juice or smoothie and abundant seasonal fruit (Preferably low-glycemic fruits: berries or stone fruits)

Midday meal   Your choice of:

- Fresh salad with seasonal vegetables and/or
- Blended raw soup or
- Raw entrée from Chapter 5, Section I—The Raw Food Cleanse recipes

Snacks   Only eat a snack if you are truly hungry. Otherwise, wait until your next meal. Your choice of:

- Fresh fruit
- Snack/side from Chapter 5, Section I—The Raw Food Cleanse
- Fresh vegetable juice
- Herbal tea
- Ecstatic Elixir
- Smart Cocktail
- Balancing Broth (page 76)

Evening meal   Your choice of:

- Smart Cocktail, Ecstatic Elixir or veggie juice and
- Fresh seasonal salad and/or
- Blended raw soup and/or
- Entrée from Chapter 5, Section I—The Raw Food Cleanse

It is perfectly suitable to exchange any meal with a quart of freshly pressed vegetable juice.

During the 7-Day Rejuvenation Cleanse, desserts are discouraged; however, a few lower-glycemic suggestions have been made in the dessert section of Chapter 5, Section I—The Raw Food Cleanse.

14-Day Deep Detox Cleanse

This 14-day cleanse is suggested when one has a bit more weight to release and when a shorter cleanse has already been successfully accomplished with good results. This cleanse is more of a commitment as the first seven days are exclusively liquids. It is still completely reasonable to complete this cleanse while working, managing a family and living your life. There is a bit more planning involved, but only because of the length of this cleanse.

During the first five days, it will be important to consume a gallon of recommended liquids daily. This is so that you won't become hungry, feel weak or have challenging detox symptoms. The first fresh juices each day can be made upon arising in the morning and stored in an airtight container in the refrigerator until you are ready to drink them. Freshly press your final evening juice right before drinking to receive the most nutritional benefit, as fresh juice loses vital life energy rather quickly. Always consume juice within 24 hours after extraction for best results and freshest flavor.

On Day 6 you will begin to introduce fiber back into your diet through Green Smoothies, blended salads and soups. During Days 8–14 you'll be on a very high raw food diet that will facilitate deep detox, bringing a renewed level of energy, well-being and weight loss.

Every day upon waking, be sure to drink 32 ounces of pure, clean water, with lemon or lime if desired.

Days 1–5

Morning meal   32-ounce fresh fruit/vegetable juice

Lunch meal   32-ounce fresh vegetable juice

Mid-afternoon meal   32-ounce fresh fruit/vegetable juice

Evening meal   32-ounce fresh vegetable juice

Herbal teas, Smart Cocktails, Ecstatic Elixirs and Balancing Broth are also allowed as desired.

Days 6–7

Morning meal   32-ounce green smoothie or fruit smoothie

Lunch meal   32-ounce smoothie or blended soup

Mid-afternoon meal   32-ounce smoothie, blended soup or blended salad

Evening meal   32-ounce blended soup or blended salad

Again, herbal teas, Smart Cocktails, Ecstatic Elixirs and Balancing Broth are also allowed as desired.

Days 8–14

Morning meal   Your choice of:

- 32-ounce Raw Cleanse juice or
- 32-ounce Raw Cleanse smoothie or
- 16-ounce juice or smoothie and abundant seasonal fruit (Preferably low-glycemic fruits: berries or stone fruits)

Midday meal   Your choice of:

- Fresh salad with seasonal vegetables and/or
- Blended raw soup or
- Raw entrée from Chapter 5, Section I—The Raw Food Cleanse

Snacks   Your choice of:

- Fresh fruit
- Cut veggies with seed cheese or hummus
- Fresh vegetable juice
- Herbal tea
- Smart Cocktail
- Ecstatic Elixir
- Balancing Broth (see page 76)

Evening meal   Your choice of:

- Smart Cocktail, Ecstatic Elixir or veggie juice and
- Fresh seasonal salad and/or
- Blended raw soup and/or
- Raw entrée from Chapter 5, Section II—Maintaining Your Cleanse for Life

It is always perfectly suitable to exchange any meal with a quart of freshly pressed vegetable juice.

Low-glycemic desserts are allowed sparingly toward the end of the 14-Day Deep Detox, if desired. See the dessert recipes in Chapter 5.

28-Day Total Body Reset Cleanse

The 28-Day Total Body Reset Cleanse is designed for those individuals who have the most weight to lose and for those with a significant background of compromised diet, unhealthy lifestyle and environmental exposures.

In this particular cleanse you will be consuming a liquid diet for the first 10–14 days. As with the other cleanse protocols, there are not many sweet fruits as they can interfere with weight loss and trigger cravings in many people. Once you have completed the 28 days, you are free to begin to enjoy all of the foods/recipes that appear in Chapter 5, Section II—Maintaining Your Cleanse for Life.

As with the other cleanses, the 28-day protocol should include the lifestyle adjustments detailed in Chapter 7 to facilitate your cleansing and detoxing.

Days 1–7

This can safely be extended to 10 days if you have a large amount of weight to lose.

Morning meal   32-ounce fresh fruit/vegetable juice

Lunch meal   32-ounce fresh vegetable juice

Mid-afternoon meal   32-ounce fresh fruit/vegetable juice

Evening meal   32-ounce fresh vegetable juice

Herbal teas, Smart Cocktails, Ecstatic Elixirs and Balancing Broth are also allowed as desired.

Days 8–10

This schedule can be followed on Days 11–14 if you are extending the liquid-diet portion of the cleanse.

Morning meal 32-ounce green smoothie or fruit smoothie

Lunch meal 32-ounce smoothie or blended soup

Mid-afternoon meal 32-ounce smoothie, blended soup or blended salad

Evening meal 32-ounce blended soup or blended salad

Again, herbal teas, Smart Cocktails, Ecstatic Elixirs and Balancing Broth are also allowed as desired.

Days 11–19

Morning meal Your choice of:
- 32-ounce Raw Cleanse juice or
- 32-ounce Raw Cleanse smoothie or
- 16-ounce juice or smoothie and abundant seasonal fruit (preferably low-glycemic fruits: berries or stone fruits)

Midday meal Your choice of:
- Fresh salad with seasonal vegetables and/or
- Blended raw soup or
- Raw entrée from Chapter 5, Section I—The Raw Food Cleanse

Evening meal Your choice of:
- Veggie juice and

- Fresh seasonal salad and/or
- Blended raw soup
- Raw entrée from Chapter 5, Section I—The Raw Food Cleanse

Snacking and desserts are discouraged during this period. If you find that you are feeling hungry, it is suitable to have fresh green vegetable juice, herbal teas, Smart Cocktails, Ecstatic Elixirs or Balancing Broth. Remember, the more greens you consume, the less you will experience cravings.

Days 20–28

Morning meal   Your choice of:

- 32-ounce Raw Cleanse juice or
- 32-ounce Raw Cleanse smoothie or
- 16-ounce juice or smoothie and abundant seasonal fruit (preferably low-glycemic fruits: berries or stone fruits)

Midday meal   Your choice of:

- Fresh salad with seasonal vegetables and/or
- Blended soup or
- Entrée from Chapter 5, Section I—The Raw Food Cleanse

Snacks   Your choice of:

- Fresh fruit or
- Cut veggies with seed cheese or hummus
- Fresh vegetable juice
- Herbal tea
- Smart Cocktail
- Ecstatic Elixir
- Balancing Broth (page 76)

Evening meal   Your choice of:

- Smart Cocktail, Ecstatic Elixir or veggie juice and
- Fresh seasonal salad and/or
- Blended soup
- Entrée from Chapter 5, Section I—The Raw Food Cleanse
- Raw Cleanse dessert, if desired

As always, it is perfectly suitable to exchange any meal with a quart of freshly pressed vegetable juice.

5

Life Cleanse Recipes

In this chapter you'll find two sections of recipes. The recipes in Section I are recommended for use during any of the four Raw Food Cleanses outlined in Chapter 4. Section II offers recipes that are healthy additions for a long-term raw food lifestyle.

Section I—The Raw Food Cleanse Recipes

Raw Food Cleanse Juices

Green Drink

1 bunch of leafy green lettuce
½ head celery
1 cucumber
1–2 Granny Smith apples, cored
1 lime, peeled

Push all ingredients through your juicer. Consume until satisfied.

My Daily Green

Spinach is one of the easiest greens to start with when juicing because of its mild flavor. It also is high in iron and coenzyme Q10. Celery has an abundance of organic sodium, of which most people are painfully deficient. Cucumber is an important player in beautifying the skin, and parsley is an intestinal purifier and deodorizer.

2 cups fresh spinach
6 stalks celery
1 medium cucumber
½ bunch flat-leaf parsley

Run all ingredients through your juicer and enjoy.

Garden Variety

A tall glass of this dark-green goodness will do your body right.

6 stalks celery
4 leaves kale
Large handful of spinach
Handful of parsley
Small handful of arugula
1 small cucumber
2 lemons, peeled

Green juices such as this are easily made in a blender. Just add ½ cup water first and start with one stalk of celery. Blend on high for 10 seconds and then add everything else. Blend, then pour into a nut-milk bag to strain.

Get Lucky Green Juice

6–8 leaves romaine

Handful of dandelion greens

6 stalks celery

½ cucumber

2–3 Granny Smith apples

1 lime, peeled

Push all ingredients through a juicer; enjoy!

Liquid Salad

In addition to being super-nutritious, this juice is really delicious and savory. The name says it all.

¼ head green leaf lettuce

¼ head purple romaine

4 stalks celery

3 carrots

2 radishes with tops

3 scallions

½ large cucumber

½ pint cherry tomatoes

2 cloves garlic

1 lemon, peeled

½ teaspoon Himalayan sea salt

Run all ingredients through your juicer. Taste, then add a bit of extra sea salt if needed to bring out the flavor.

Green Beauty

This juice is one of the best combinations for cleansing and beautifying. The organic sodium of celery helps to transport the water- and silica-rich cucumber juice into your body's tissues, which creates super hydration.

6 stalks celery

1 small cucumber

Handful of spinach (or other leafy green)

1 large apple

Run all ingredients through a juicer. Serve over ice in a tall glass for ultimate beautification!

Spring Green Goodness

This juice was inspired by a bountiful trip to a late-spring farmers' market.

1 large cucumber

1 small head Boston/Bibb/butter lettuce

2 shallots

2 radishes with tops

2 stalks fresh spring garlic

2 limes, peeled

1 tablespoon raw local honey, or to taste

Push the first six ingredients through a juicer, then mix in honey to taste.

Pico de Gallo

Ease your Mexican food craving with this spicy little number!

4 stalks celery

6 leaves romaine

1 small bunch cilantro

1 small red bell pepper

1 pint cherry tomatoes

2 carrots

½ small sweet onion

3 cloves garlic

1 jalapeño
2 limes, peeled
Pinch of Himalayan sea salt
A good splash of apple cider vinegar

Push all fruits and vegetables through a juicer, then blend a pinch of sea salt and a splash of apple cider vinegar into the finished juice.

Thai Green Transfusion

The idea for this juice was born during a trip to the local Asian market.

6 stalks celery
Handful of sugar snap peas
½ cup alfalfa sprouts
3 scallions
½ red bell pepper
2 serrano chiles
½ pint cherry tomatoes
½ bunch cilantro
2 limes, peeled
Water of one young coconut
2 teaspoons flaxseed oil
Celtic sea salt, to taste

Juice all ingredients up to the coconut. Transfer the liquid to a blender; add the young coconut water, flaxseed oil and salt, and blend until smooth.

Spicy Green Tomato

I tried to create a juice that tasted like the popular commercial brand, keeping it as close to the original combination of eight ingredients as possible without sacrificing taste. This is a powerhouse of live nutrition!

1 pint grape tomatoes

6 stalks celery

4 carrots

Handful of spinach

1/3 bunch cilantro

Handful of arugula

2 cloves garlic

1 jalapeño

2 lemons, peeled

1 tablespoon olive oil

1 tablespoon raw honey

Celtic sea salt and freshly ground black pepper, to taste

Juice all the fruits and vegetables. Pour into a blender
and add the oil, honey, salt and pepper, then blend
well until a bit emulsified (about 20 seconds).

My Green Goddess

*Depending on how sweet or tart you want this juice to
taste, you can change up the variety of apple.*

1 small bunch lacinato kale or baby spinach

4 celery stalks

1 organic lemon, peeled

1 small bunch flat leaf parsley

1-inch piece fresh ginger

2 apples, variety of choice

Push all ingredients through a juicer. Drink
immediately.

Stone Temple Purifier

Stone fruits create a low-glycemic taste sensation.

2 large apricots, pitted

3 ripe peaches, pitted

1 cup fresh cherries, seeded

1 lemon, peeled

1 teaspoon ginseng powder (optional)

Push all ingredients through a juicer. This can also be a delicious smoothie if you prefer to add all ingredients to your blender for a thicker drink.

Green Mechanic

This is the perfect tune-up for your engine— guaranteed to kick out any unwanted cobwebs.

½ head celery

3 Granny Smith apples

2 cups alfalfa sprouts

½ bunch parsley

Handful of mint leaves

1 lime, peeled

Juice all ingredients, pour into a tall glass and enjoy.

Green Gringo

This was my favorite juice nearly every night for at least a month while on my three-month juice feast. It really satisfied my taste memory for Mexican food!

6 stalks celery

Handful of spinach

5 scallions

1 pint cherry tomatoes

Small bunch cilantro

1–2 jalapeños

2 cloves garlic

1 lime, peeled

1 tablespoon apple cider vinegar

Sea salt and freshly cracked black pepper to taste

Juice all ingredients except the apple cider vinegar, salt and pepper. Add those to the finished juice by stirring in before drinking. This juice is especially refreshing served over ice.

Purple Passion

Cabbage, with its natural antibacterial properties; apples, with their natural ability to cleanse; and celery, with its re-mineralizing capabilities, make for a surprisingly delicious, colorful juice.

½ small red cabbage
2 stalks celery
2 apples
1 tablespoon fresh lemon juice

Chop the cabbage and apples and feed all ingredients through a juicer. Serve immediately.

Berries Unite

This multi-berry, orange and sea-algae combo is the bomb. This is a juice that contains lots of vitamin C and antioxidants galore. It's also an immune booster, and drinking it regularly may decrease the risk of developing certain cancers. Oranges are rich in folic acid and potassium, while berries pack a calcium punch for healthy bones and teeth. This combo is also thought to help soothe the nervous system.

1 pint fresh organic strawberries
½ pint fresh raspberries
½ pint fresh blueberries
4 oranges, peeled
½ cup Thai coconut water
1 tablespoon Crystal Manna Flakes

You can choose to either juice or blend the berries. I generally use a Vita-Mix to blend, then I strain the combination through a nut-milk bag to remove the pulp and seeds, but it is perfectly fine to leave them in if you choose. Once you have a smooth, clear liquid, pour back into your clean blender and add a bit of crushed ice, re-blending to the consistency of a smoothie. A delicious treat!

Island Flush

The powerful protein-digesting enzymes in pineapple help to clean up the digestive tract by breaking down and "digesting" dead cells, which actually helps heal damaged digestive systems. This wonder fruit also purifies the blood and helps clear excess mucus buildup. Paired with cilantro, a widely known heavy-metal detoxifier, this drink rolls up its sleeves and gets down to business!

½ small pineapple, peeled, cored and sliced
1 small handful cilantro
4 stalks celery
1 lime, peeled
2 apples
Push all ingredients through a juicer and enjoy.

One Hot Ruby

4 cups watermelon juice (about ½ medium watermelon)
1 lime, peeled
¾-inch piece ginger, grated

Juice the watermelon and lime, pour into your blender and whirl with the grated ginger for a great morning wake-up call!

Raw Food Cleanse Smoothies & Shakes

THE Green Smoothie

2 big handfuls of spinach or kale (de-veined)

1 cup fresh or frozen berries

1 teaspoon coconut oil

1 tablespoon chia seeds, soaked

2 cups of fresh almond milk or water

Place all ingredients in your blender and combine until smooth and creamy.

Wild Thing

Dandelion greens are nutritious—high in vitamin A, vitamin C and iron. They're also low in calories, fat and cholesterol. Plus, wild greens are widely available and require no work at all—except harvesting! As with any green, the younger the plant, the more tender it is. For the safest crop, be sure to pick greens well away from major roads or other chemically treated areas, and wash the greens thoroughly before you use them.

Handful of dandelion greens

Handful of flat-leaf parsley

Handful of spinach

1 frozen banana

1 orange, peeled and in segments

1 cup frozen raspberries

Combine all ingredients in a blender.

Gentle Liver-Cleanse Smoothie

4 cups fresh wild greens (dandelion, lamb's quarters, purslane)

½ head curly endive

1 cup cilantro

2 cups apple juice, fresh

1 banana

2 pears

½-inch piece ginger

1 cup cranberries

Blend well—and don't go on a road trip right after you drink it. (Hee hee.)

Chia Coconut Custard Shake

Thank the chia seeds for making this delicious shake fall into the low-glycemic category! This shake is allowed in all four cleanses. You must try this one.

2 young coconuts, meat and water

2 tablespoons chia seeds, soaked for 15 minutes in 1 cup water

½ cup crushed ice

¼ cup raw honey or agave nectar

2 teaspoons vanilla extract

A generous pinch each of cinnamon, nutmeg and sea salt

Put all ingredients into a high-speed blender and blend until smooth and creamy.

Berry Bliss

3 big romaine leaves

1 handful sunflower sprouts

2 handfuls baby spinach

1–10 frozen strawberries

1 handful frozen or fresh blueberries

1 cup water

2 tablespoons aloe vera juice (optional)

Blend all ingredients together until smooth and well combined.

Exotic Endurance

2 large handfuls organic spinach
2 large handfuls mixed baby greens
½ cup alfalfa sprouts
1 tablespoon chia seeds
1 tablespoon golden flaxseeds, ground
½ small pineapple, peeled, cored and sliced
1 small banana
1 cup water

Combine all ingredients in a blender until smooth.

The Charmer and the Kale

This smoothie recipe is from Heather, one of our RFC guinea pigs. For this one, she sings, "Hi-ho, the derry-o, the charmer and the kale!"

1 bunch kale
½ pineapple, peeled, cored and sliced
1 Fuji apple
2 cups strawberries
1 cup ice
½ cup water

Combine all ingredients in a blender.

Lemon Rescue

This smoothie is the perfect remedy if you suffer from seasonal allergies or feel a cold coming on.

1 young coconut, meat and milk
3 organic lemons, peeled

1 teaspoon lemon zest
2 tablespoons raw honey (local honey is best)
Small piece of fresh ginger (grated)
Pinch of cayenne pepper

Combine all ingredients in a blender until smooth and creamy.

Fruit 'n' Fiber

Never underestimate the power of a little fiber!

1 frozen banana
½ cup blueberries
Handful of strawberries
2 tablespoons golden flaxseeds, ground
Small handful of goji berries
½ cup fresh almond milk
½ cup water, to thin

Blend all ingredients until smooth.

Raspberry Love

1 pint fresh or frozen raspberries
2 ripe pears
2 handfuls of spinach
2 cups chilled water

Combine ingredients and blend until smooth.

Goji High

1 cup frozen or fresh blueberries
Handful goji berries, soaked for 15 minutes
1 cup vanilla hemp milk
1 cup ice

Combine ingredients in a blender.

Katie's Coconut Chia Fruit Smoothie

2 tablespoons dehydrated coconut
2 tablespoons chia seeds
1 large juicing orange, peeled
½ cup frozen strawberries
½ cup ice
Vanilla bean powder or vanilla extract to taste
Stevia and honey to taste

Blend all ingredients together. Pour into a glass and top with blueberries or goji berries.

Blueberry Hemp-Nut Shake

With the high protein and essential fatty acids of hemp nuts and the powerful antioxidant superfood status of blueberries, this shake won't let you down. Hemp nuts make a fantastic base for smoothies or shakes because they don't need to be pre-soaked. Since they're already soft, when blended they instantly become a creamy milk that needs no straining. The milk will be white with dark specks that look like blended vanilla bean.

2 cups pure water
½ cup hemp nuts (seeds)
3 tablespoons agave nectar
1 teaspoon vanilla extract or raw vanilla powder
1 small package frozen blueberries
1 frozen banana
Pinch of sea salt

Start by putting the water and hemp nuts in a blender and processing until well blended. Add the agave nectar, vanilla, blueberries, frozen banana and salt, and blend into a smooth, creamy, yummy shake.

Raw Food Cleanse Smart Cocktails

THE Smart Cocktail

½ cup kombucha
⅓ cup fresh fruit juice of choice
Juice from lemon or lime wedges (to taste)
Sparkling mineral water

Mix the kombucha and fresh fruit juice and pour into a
tall glass filled with ice. Squeeze in the lemon or lime
juice and top off with sparkling mineral water.

Virgin Mary

6 large ripe tomatoes
1 lemon, peeled
4 stalks celery
2 teaspoons nama shoyu
¼ teaspoon freshly ground nutmeg
¼ teaspoon cayenne pepper
Celtic sea salt and freshly cracked black pepper to taste

Juice the tomatoes, lemon and 3 stalks of the celery.
Pour into a blender and add nama shoyu, nutmeg,
cayenne, and salt and pepper, then blend just long
enough to incorporate. Pour the mixture over crushed
ice in a tall glass; serve with a celery stalk and a
lemon twist.

Razzle Dazzle

1 pint fresh raspberries (frozen is also fine)
6 Granny Smith or other tart, low-glycemic variety of apples
⅓ cup sparkling mineral water
Mint sprigs for garnish

Push the raspberries and apples through your juicer. Pour into a small pitcher and add sparkling water; stir to combine. Pour over ice in pretty glasses and garnish with a sprig of mint.

Ginger-Peach Bellini

2-inch piece ginger, sliced into thin rounds
¼ cup water
¼ cup agave nectar
1 cup peaches, peeled and sliced
1 bottle GT's Organic Raw Kombucha
Additional peach slices for garnish

In a small saucepan, combine the ginger and water. Steep over medium heat for about 10 minutes, then strain the ginger water, immediately stirring in the agave nectar to create a simple ginger syrup. Once cooled, pour the syrup and peaches into a blender and blend until smooth. Pour purée into the bottom of a champagne glass and top with kombucha. Garnish each glass with a peach slice.

Healthy Hound

A nonalcoholic version of the Greyhound.

½ cup grapefruit juice
½ cup GT's Organic Raw Kombucha (can substitute sparkling water)
½ lime, juiced
1 tablespoon raw honey (can use agave nectar)
Handful fresh mint leaves, chopped

If you own a citrus press, this drink is a no-brainer. You can also squeeze the grapefruit by hand. Mix the grapefruit juice, kombucha, lime juice, sweetener and mint in a small pitcher. Serve in a pretty glass over ice.

Raw Food Cleanse Ecstatic Elixirs

The Rubyvroom

My friend, the talented raw food chef Frank Giglio, created this elixir in my honor after an inspiration during a morning run. If you don't have a copy of Frank's 2009 collection of raw recipes, Raw For All, *you'll want to be sure to get the hookup on that. (See the Resources section for more information.)*

1½ cups hibiscus tea, chilled

Seeds of 1 pomegranate (about ¾ cup)

1 cup frozen strawberries

Pinch of cayenne (more or less, depending on sassiness!)

½ lime, peeled

1 teaspoon honey

1 teaspoon royal jelly

4 sprays of rose hydrosol (see the Resources section for recommended retailers)

Blend well, and enjoy!

Citrus Basil Infusion

Basil brings a subtle herbal note to this interesting citrus-berry infusion.

4 large basil sprigs (about ½ cup firmly packed), plus more for garnish

⅔ cup agave nectar

2 large limes, juiced

1 large lemon, juiced

1 medium orange, juiced

2 tablespoons frozen raspberries
1 cup sparkling mineral water

In a saucepan, gently steep basil leaves in ⅓ cup water on low heat for about 30 minutes. Remove from heat and stir in agave nectar. Allow to cool to room temperature, then strain, pressing on the basil leaves to release more flavor. Pour lime, lemon and orange juices into a blender along with the strained basil syrup. Blend until smooth, and strain into a pitcher. Stir in sparkling mineral water. Pour into glasses over ice and serve with basil sprigs.

Yerba Latte

Yerba maté is a medicinal and cultural drink with ancient origins. Maté contains ingredients that are believed to keep its drinkers healthy and energetic. The tea is a cultural phenomenon throughout South America, where the sight of an obese person is rare. Although I've technically given up caffeine this year, I occasionally live on the edge and have a cup of maté as a delicious raw-food-friendly latte.

2 tablespoons dried loose yerba maté tea leaves
1-inch piece fresh ginger, sliced
1 stick cinnamon
½ vanilla bean
¼ teaspoon grated nutmeg
1 cup honey-sweetened Brazil-nut milk

Place the tea leaves in 2 cups of water in a medium saucepan and brew gently over low heat for a few minutes. Once steeped, place the ginger, cinnamon, nutmeg and vanilla bean into the warm tea and continue to steep on very low heat for about 5–10 minutes. Strain the mixture and blend equal parts tea and nut milk to create the latte. Sprinkle with freshly grated nutmeg and serve warm in a heated mug.

Rosie Rooibos

Rooibos tea is one of my favorite herbal teas. It comes from the stems and leaves of a woody legume grown in South Africa's Western Cape Province. It's low in tannins, caffeine free and loaded with antioxidants and other healing agents.

5 large rosemary sprigs
1½ teaspoons rooibos tea leaves
½ cup agave nectar
4 tablespoons fresh lemon juice
1 cup kombucha

In a small saucepan, steep rosemary sprigs in one cup of water for 10 minutes over low heat. Add in rooibos tea and allow to steep over very low heat for one hour. Remove from heat and add agave nectar, allowing flavors to marry for another 15 minutes. Strain through a fine-mesh sieve and discard tea leaves and rosemary.

Mix the rooibos-rosemary infusion with lemon juice in a cocktail shaker filled with ice cubes. Pour equal parts infusion and kombucha into ice-filled glasses, garnish with fresh rosemary sprigs and serve.

Lemony Licorice

1 tablespoon dried licorice tea leaves
1 tablespoon dried spearmint leaves
Handful of fresh basil leaves
Lemon wedges

Place licorice and spearmint into a teapot. Muddle the basil leaves a bit first to release their flavor, then add them to the pot. Fill the pot with 4 cups of hot water, cover, and steep about three to five minutes. Strain into warm mugs, garnishing with basil leaves and lemon wedges. If the licorice is too strong for you, just add lemon juice.

Raw Food Cleanse Dressings & Sauces

Cilantro Lime Dressing

1 cup fresh cilantro
½ cup extra virgin olive oil
¼ cup fresh lime juice
¼ cup fresh orange juice
1 teaspoon lime zest
½ teaspoon sea salt
½ teaspoon freshly ground black pepper
Pinch of minced garlic

Purée cilantro, olive oil, lime juice, orange juice, lime zest, salt, pepper and garlic in a blender or food processor until smooth.

Creamy Macadamia Dressing

¾ cup macadamia nuts, soaked for at least an hour
1 teaspoon orange zest
1 teaspoon ground cumin
⅛ teaspoon sea salt
Pinch of cayenne pepper

Place the drained macadamia nuts into a blender with ¼ cup water. Add the other ingredients and blend until creamy. Add more water, if necessary—half a teaspoon at a time—to thin out as desired. As with all nut-based dressings, use sparingly.

Thai Salad Dressing

2 cloves garlic, minced
1 red chile, de-seeded and minced
1 tablespoon namu shoyu
Juice of ½ lime (about 1 tablespoon)
2 teaspoons agave nectar
1 tablespoon pineapple juice (optional)

Blend all ingredients in a blender until creamy.

"Thousand Island"

2 oranges, peeled and seeded
4 tablespoons olive oil
2 tablespoons raw honey
2 tablespoons nama shoyu
¼ cup raw almond or cashew butter
2 tablespoons apple cider vinegar or fresh lemon juice
4 cloves garlic

You can use a food processor or blender to make this creamy dressing.

French Dressing

½ cup water or Balancing Broth (page 76)
⅓ cup fresh lemon juice
1 tablespoon paprika
1 clove garlic
¾ cup Roma tomatoes, seeds removed
⅓ cup raw honey

1 tablespoon chopped sweet onion

½ teaspoon sea salt

In your blender, combine all ingredients until well emulsified. Store in an airtight container in the refrigerator. Keeps well for one week if water was used, or for several days if broth was used.

Raw Mustard

½ cup mustard seeds

½ cup mineral water

6 tablespoons fresh lemon juice

2 tablespoons raw honey or agave nectar

Soak the seeds in water and lemon juice overnight. Add honey and blend in a food processor or blender until creamy. Will keep for months in the fridge.

Honey Mustard Dressing

½ cup Raw Mustard (see above)

½ cup olive oil

½ cup raw honey or agave nectar

½ cup water (less water will make for a creamier dressing)

Blend all ingredients well.

Stacey's Lemon Tahini Dressing or Dip

½ cup olive oil

⅔ cup lemon juice

⅓ cup wheat-free tamari

1 cup tahini

¼ cup diced red bell pepper

⅓ cup diced onion

2 stalks celery

¼ cup parsley

½ tablespoon agave nectar

Blend all ingredients until smooth. If too thick, add water (up to ¼ cup) until dressing pours (or keep thick to use as a dip). If too bitter, add lemon juice and more agave nectar. Will keep in fridge in an airtight container for two weeks.

Tahini Dressing 2.0

1 cup raw tahini

¾ cup olive oil

⅔ cup fresh orange juice

3 cloves garlic

1½ inches fresh ginger

1 tablespoon nama shoyu

1–2 teaspoons dulse or kelp granules

¼ cup fresh cilantro

Blend all ingredients together until creamy and well combined. This is wonderful on a salad, in an Asian slaw or stir-fry, or with nori rolls.

Raw Food Cleanse Spectacular Salads

Any of these salads can be eaten as is or blended into a liquid consistency for easier assimilation.

Fiesta Salad

Mixed greens

Fresh tomatoes, chopped

Red onion, thinly sliced

Orange bell pepper, chopped

Onion sprouts
Avocado, cubed

Use amounts of each ingredient to your liking. Dress
with Cilantro Lime Dressing (page 65).

Good Vibrations Salad

Lettuce greens of choice
Dulse, crumbled
Carrot, grated
Cucumber, chopped
Cherry tomatoes
Sprouts
Hemp seeds

Use amounts of each ingredient to your liking
and dress with Creamy Macadamia Dressing (page 66).

Orange Spinach Salad
with Orange Tahini Dressing

This is a classic and a favorite at my house.

For the salad:
4 cups fresh baby spinach leaves
½ cup fresh baby bella mushrooms, sliced
1 orange, peeled and sliced
⅓ cup red onion, finely sliced
⅓ cup walnuts

For the dressing:
1 cup fresh orange juice
Small handful of pitted dates
¼ cup raw tahini
2 cloves garlic

1 teaspoon lemon zest

1 tablespoon fresh lemon juice

Make the dressing first by placing all the ingredients in a blender and mixing until emulsified. Toss the spinach, mushrooms, orange and red onion in the dressing and assemble the salad on a plate. Top with pieces of raw walnut.

Wild Greek Salad

For the salad:

2 cups lamb's quarters (greens)

2 cucumbers, sliced

2 tomatoes, diced

¼ cup red onion, finely sliced

⅓ cup raw olives

2 teaspoons fresh oregano (try to use tender, young leaves for this salad)

For the dressing:

1½ tablespoons lemon juice, freshly squeezed

1½ tablespoons apple cider vinegar

1 clove garlic

½ cup cold-pressed extra virgin olive oil

¾ teaspoon sea salt

2 tablespoons fresh herbs of choice (e.g., dill, parsley, oregano)

¼ teaspoon freshly cracked black pepper

Blend the dressing ingredients in a blender until smooth. Coat salad just before serving.

Fresh Corn & Tomato Salad

3 ears fresh corn, kernels cut from the cob

2 Roma tomatoes, diced

1 small red bell pepper, diced
¼ cup diced red onion
1–2 cloves fresh garlic, minced
¼ cup chopped cilantro
1 lime, juiced
½ lemon, juiced
Drizzle of extra virgin olive oil
Sea salt and freshly ground black pepper to taste

Combine all ingredients and chill before serving.

Garden-Fresh Chilled Summer Salad

This is a refrigerator staple at our house in the summer.

1 pint cherry or other small tomatoes
1 large cucumber
1 large sweet summer onion
Handful fresh garden herbs, chopped
½ cup apple cider or rice wine vinegar
1 lemon, juiced
2 tablespoons raw honey
Sea salt and freshly ground black pepper to taste

Halve the tomatoes. Halve the cucumber lengthwise, then remove seeds from the center and slice into half-moon pieces about ⅛-inch thick. Halve the onion and slice finely, leaving in half-rings.

Combine the remaining ingredients to make the marinade and pour over the vegetables to thoroughly coat. Chill for an hour before serving.

Marinated Asparagus

1 bunch fresh asparagus
3 tablespoons red wine vinegar
2 tablespoons stone-ground mustard

1 tablespoon fresh lemon juice

3 tablespoons olive oil

1 teaspoon sea salt

Freshly ground black pepper to taste

Chopped fresh parsley or chives for garnish

Lemon zest for garnish

Trim off the tough ends from the asparagus. Whisk together the remaining ingredients (except garnish) in a small bowl to make the marinade. Place the asparagus in a zippered plastic bag and pour the marinade over it, using your hands to incorporate and cover fully. Store in the refrigerator. Plate up and garnish when ready to serve.

Janine's Pineapple Thai Salad

1 to 1½ cups fresh pineapple chunks

1 English cucumber or medium field cucumber, cut in chunks

1 red bell pepper, sliced thinly or diced

3 spring onions (green onions), sliced

½ cup raw nuts, roughly chopped

1 cup fresh cilantro

Handful of fresh basil leaves (roughly chopped if leaves are large)

Ground or chopped nuts and lime wedges for garnish

Place pineapple chunks, cucumber chunks, red bell pepper, green onion and nuts in a mixing bowl. Add most of the cilantro and basil, setting aside a little of each for the garnish. Toss well with Thai Salad Dressing (page 66). Place salad onto a serving plate and garnish with reserved basil and cilantro, plus a sprinkling of ground or chopped nuts. If desired, serve with lime wedges on the side.

Note: This salad is at its best when first tossed. Try to eat up leftovers as soon as possible.

Pineapple-Jalapeño Coleslaw

¼ cup fresh pineapple juice

¼ cup seasoned rice vinegar (or substitute apple cider vinegar)

1½ tablespoons flaxseed or olive oil

1 tablespoon agave nectar

3 tablespoons chopped jalapeño pepper

1 teaspoon lime zest

½ teaspoon coarse sea salt

6 cups thinly sliced napa (Chinese) cabbage

2 cups grated peeled jicama

1 cup grated peeled carrot

¾ cup thinly sliced green onions

¼ cup chopped fresh cilantro

¼ cup chopped fresh mint

Combine first seven ingredients in a small bowl, stirring with a whisk. Combine cabbage and remaining ingredients in a large bowl. Pour dressing over cabbage mixture; toss gently to coat. Serve immediately.

Asian Cucumber Salad

3 tablespoons fresh lime juice

2 tablespoons nama shoyu or wheat-free tamari

1 tablespoon maple syrup or agave nectar

1 clove fresh minced garlic

1 tablespoon fresh mint, roughly chopped

1 teaspoon seeded, minced jalapeño pepper (or more
   to taste)
2 large cucumbers, sliced lengthwise on a mandoline or
   with a sharp knife to about ⅛-inch thickness
¼ cup raw peanuts, chopped

In a small bowl, mix lime juice, nama shoyu, maple
syrup, garlic, mint and jalapeño. Add cucumber
ribbons and peanuts, tossing gently. Serve within
one hour.

Raw Marinated Vegetable Salad

For the salad (amounts as desired):
Mushrooms, sliced
Red bell pepper, julienned
Tomatoes, diced
Sun-dried tomatoes (soaked 1 hour), diced
Red onion, finely sliced
Parsley, chopped
Rosemary, chopped
Basil, chopped

For the marinade:
Lemon juice
Nama shoyu (or wheat-free tamari)
Olive oil
Fresh garlic, minced
Fresh thyme

Toss all the salad ingredients with the marinade.
Allow the flavors to marry for 30 minutes to an hour
before serving.

Janine Gibbons' Jicama Lime Salad

1 medium jicama, peeled and chopped into ½-inch cubes
  (approximately 2 cups)
1 medium cucumber, peeled and seeded, chopped into
  ½-inch cubes (approximately 1½ cups)
1 small lime, juice and zest
½–1 teaspoon sea salt (to taste)
⅛ teaspoon dried chipotle powder or chili powder
Dash cayenne pepper

In a medium-size bowl, mix all the ingredients
together. Let stand at room temperature for 1 hour to
allow the flavors to blend.

Marinated Broccoli

4 cups broccoli florets
⅓ cup fresh oregano
⅓ cup fresh basil
½ cup olive oil
¼ cup fresh lemon juice
¼ cup red bell pepper, chopped
1 clove garlic, minced

Combine ingredients and marinate all day in the
refrigerator. If you have a dehydrator, this dish is extra
delicious when heated in the dehydrator for about an
hour at 115 degrees.

Raw Food Cleanse Soups

Except for Balancing Broth, these soups can be served at room temperature, chilled, or warmed in your high-speed blender.

Balancing Broth

Although cooked, this vegetable broth is very grounding and nutritious as a base for soups. It can also be consumed on its own. Being able to have something warm helps many people as they begin transitioning to a high raw food diet. I recommend keeping some of this on hand throughout all of the four cleanses. Please try to buy only organic vegetables for this soup.

2 onions, scrubbed, skin left on

4 carrots, not peeled

4 stalks celery

2 potatoes, any variety, scrubbed, skin on

2 cups broccoli

4 cloves garlic, crushed

½ cup fresh chopped parsley

2 bay leaves

1½-inch piece kombu seaweed

1 teaspoon each fresh thyme and basil (dried is also fine)

Pinch of cayenne, if desired

Chop the onions, carrots, celery, potatoes and broccoli into 1-inch cubes. Place in a stock pot, add remaining ingredients, cover with 10 cups pure filtered water and bring to a boil. Continue cooking over low heat for one hour. Cool, strain, discard the vegetables and store broth in an airtight container (glass Mason jars are great) in your refrigerator. Keeps well for about one week, or you can freeze.

Market Fresh Tomato Soup

1 quart fresh tomatoes

2 shallots

½ bunch basil

3 stalks celery

Handful of fresh oregano

2 cloves garlic

1 tablespoon olive oil

Juice of ½ lemon

1 tablespoon local raw honey, to taste

Place all ingredients into a high-speed blender and mix until smooth and creamy.

Creamy Avocado Soup

2 avocados, peeled and pitted

2½ tablespoons miso, brown or white

2 tablespoons olive oil

Juice of 1 lime

1 teaspoon fresh rosemary, or other fresh herb of your choice

½ teaspoon dried chipotle (optional)

2–3 cups pure water (depending on how thick you want the soup to be)

Diced tomatoes for garnish

Blend all ingredients in your blender until well combined and creamy. Sprinkle diced tomatoes on top and serve.

Herb-ocado

2 handfuls of mixed greens

1 large avocado, peeled and pitted

¼ cup lemon juice

3–4 tablespoons fresh parsley

3–4 tablespoons fresh oregano

3–4 tablespoons fresh thyme

1 tablespoon Bragg Liquid Aminos (optional)

¼ cup extra virgin olive oil

Sea salt and freshly ground black pepper to taste

1 cup filtered water, or more to reach desired consistency

Blend all ingredients in a high-speed blender until smooth and creamy.

Liquid Gazpacho

4 cups fresh tomato juice

⅔ cup filtered water or vegetable stock

⅔ cup peeled, seeded, and diced cucumber

⅔ cup corn, fresh or frozen

½ cup diced red bell pepper

⅓ cup diced red onion

3 tablespoons fresh lime juice

3 tablespoons minced cilantro

1 tablespoon nama shoyu, or to taste

1 tablespoon minced basil

1¼ teaspoons cumin powder

1 teaspoon minced garlic

1 teaspoon seeded and minced jalapeño pepper

½ teaspoon chili powder

Pinch of cayenne pepper

Sea salt and freshly ground black pepper, to taste

The ingredients for this soup can be chopped

and served chunky or blended into a smooth, creamy consistency.

Tomatillo Salsa Verde

1 pound tomatillos, husked
1 jalapeño (serrano chiles work well, too)
Few stalks celery
1 small Vidalia onion
1–2 lemons, peeled
2 cloves garlic
Handful of fresh cilantro
1 cup young coconut water
1 tablespoon cold-pressed olive oil, hemp oil or
    macadamia nut oil
1–2 tablespoons raw honey

Push all ingredients through your juicer except the coconut water, oil and honey. Then combine all ingredients in your Vita-Mix and blend 30 seconds, or until creamy.

Tabbouleh in a Bowl

2 cucumbers
1 bunch fresh mint
1 bunch curly leaf parsley
1 bunch scallions
1 large handful grape tomatoes
½ head romaine
2 organic lemons
1–2 cloves garlic
Celtic sea salt and freshly cracked black pepper, to taste
Hemp seeds, as garnish

This soup can be juiced, blended or chopped to suit your taste, and is best served chilled.

Chilled Cucumber Soup

This combination was created as I was preparing a cucumber salad for my family. I just started pushing some of the ingredients into my juicer and a new star was born!

6 small pickling cucumbers
Large handful of fresh dill
½ cup sugar snap peas
2 cloves garlic
½ pint onion sprouts
5 scallions
1 organic lemon, peeled
1 tablespoon olive oil
1 tablespoon apple cider vinegar
1 tablespoon raw honey
Sea salt and freshly cracked black pepper, to taste

Feed the first seven ingredients through your juicer. Pour the juice into your blender, add olive oil, vinegar, honey, salt and cracked pepper, and blend. Serve chilled and garnish with fresh peas and dill.

Thai Soup

3 carrots
1 orange bell pepper
¾ cup coconut meat (or substitute soaked cashews)
2 cups warm water
¾ cup almond milk
1 tablespoon nama shoyu
1 tablespoon agave nectar
½ jalapeño
1 tablespoon cilantro
1 tablespoon curry powder

2 teaspoons sea salt

Fresh chives, chopped, for garnish

Add all ingredients to your blender and blend until combined well.

Green Curry

This combination was inspired by a trip to my local Asian market, Nam Hai. This is seriously one of the best exotic combinations I've tried.

2 cups fresh spinach

1 small bunch fresh cilantro

½ cup young Thai coconut water

1 stalk lemongrass

1–2 Thai bird chiles

3 cloves garlic

1 thumb-size piece of fresh ginger

Juice of 2 limes

½ tablespoon ground coriander

1 teaspoon ground cumin

1 tablespoon hemp oil

1 tablespoon agave nectar

1 teaspoon nama shoyu

Juice together the spinach, fresh cilantro, coconut water, lemongrass, chiles, garlic and ginger. Pour into your blender and add the lime juice, coriander, cumin, hemp oil, agave nectar and nama shoyu. Blend until well incorporated.

Killer Summer Celery Soup

½ bunch celery

½ bunch cilantro

¼ cup water

¼ cup nut or seed butter

¼ cup raw tahini (or use more nut/seed butter)

2 small cloves garlic

2 tablespoons miso

1 tablespoon nama shoyu or wheat-free tamari

2 tablespoons lemon juice

Blend in your high-speed blender, adding ingredients slowly until the mixture is well combined and creamy. More water may be added to reach desired consistency. This soup is really delicious!

Veggie Chowder

For a thick, hearty chowder, use Killer Summer Celery Soup, above, as the base and add:

2 zucchini, grated

2 carrots, grated

1 avocado, cubed

3 ears of corn, cut kernels

1 red bell pepper, diced

Put the vegetables into the soup base, stirring gently. Slightly warm this soup for a nice fall or winter meal.

Blended Bruschetta

1 pint (or more) grape or cherry tomatoes

1 sweet Vidalia onion (you can substitute red or other variety)

1 bunch basil

2–3 cloves garlic

½ head celery

1 red bell pepper

½ large cucumber

Juice of one lemon

Celtic sea salt and freshly ground black pepper, to taste

This soup can be served blended or chopped; chilled or at room temperature.

Raw Food Cleanse Side Dishes & Snacks

Penni's Patio Salsa

Most of these ingredients can easily be grown in pots on your patio!

24 golden cherry or pear patio tomatoes

2 small heirloom tomatoes

1 serrano chile, seeded and minced

1 jalapeño, seeded and minced

3 limes, juiced

¼ cup cilantro, chopped

3 spring onions, minced

½ teaspoon sea salt

½ teaspoon freshly cracked black pepper

Blend all ingredients, then cover and refrigerate for about an hour before serving.

THE Best Guacamole

Taken from the chef's notes on my napkin while visiting the hottest Mexican restaurant in San Francisco in 1998. Still my favorite guac recipe.

2 ripe avocados

Fresh cilantro

Serrano chiles

Diced tomatoes

Fresh lime juice (be generous)

Red onions, diced
Garlic, minced
Sea salt

Amounts . . . you'll just have to figure them out like I
did. Mash avocados in a bowl and add the remaining
ingredients to taste.

Cashew Cheese

*Life just isn't worth living without some cheese. Feel
free to add in fresh chopped herbs if you desire.*

1½ cups raw cashew nuts, soaked 2 hours
2 teaspoons freshly squeezed lemon juice
2 cloves garlic, finely minced
½ teaspoon fine sea salt
Freshly ground black pepper to taste

Place the nuts in a salad bowl, cover with fresh water,
and let stand for two hours. Drain the nuts and put
them in a food processor or blender. Add ¼ cup water
and the rest of the ingredients, then mix until
thoroughly puréed, stopping to scrape the sides of the
bowl every once in a while. If necessary, add a little
more water and blend again to adjust the consistency;
the cheese will get a bit more solid as it sets.

Transfer to a bowl, cover, and let stand somewhere
cool for 24 hours before placing in the fridge, where it
will keep for another five days.

Penni's Pesto

*Use this on zucchini pasta and raw lasagna or enjoy it
on fresh tomato slices, drizzled in balsamic vinegar.*

4 cups fresh basil (you can substitute spinach if you're short
on basil)

⅓ cup olive oil

⅓ cup pine nuts

2 cloves garlic

3 tablespoons fresh lemon juice

1 tablespoon nutritional yeast (optional)

1 teaspoon sea salt

Freshly cracked black pepper to taste

Combine all ingredients in a food processor, pulsing until you achieve the desired consistency. Transfer into a small covered bowl and store in your refrigerator. This should keep for one to three days. You can also easily freeze this pesto and thaw when ready to use.

Sun & Sea Pâté

1 cup sunflower seeds (raw, soaked and sprouted)

¾ cup almonds, soaked 4 or more hours

1 stalk celery

½ bunch cilantro

1 clove garlic

¼ cup nama shoyu

¼ cup lemon juice

½ teaspoon dulse or kelp

Using a food processor, blend ingredients until smooth. This will keep well in the refrigerator for five days. Use on dehydrated crackers, carrots, celery, cucumbers, or any other veggies.

Easy Raw Hummus

1 cup sunflower seeds, soaked 1 hour

2 cups zucchini, peeled and chopped

2 cloves garlic

½ cup raw tahini

¼ cup fresh lime or lemon juice

⅓ cup water

¼ cup olive oil

2 teaspoons sea salt

Mix in a food processor or blender to create a delicious, creamy dip. You can serve with cut veggies or use as a spread for wraps.

Sun-dried Tomato & Jalapeño Hummus

Yes, we're living on the edge and using cooked chickpeas for this one.

4 cups cooked garbanzo beans

½ cup soaked and drained sun-dried tomatoes

½ cup lemon juice

3 garlic cloves, minced

¼ cup tahini

1 jalapeño pepper, veined and seeded

Blend all ingredients in a food processor, adding up to 1 cup pure water as necessary to thin.

"Roasted" Red Bell Pepper Hummus

This savory dip is best served with slices of cucumber, zucchini, bell pepper, celery stalks or carrot sticks. It is also delicious with raw onion bread or flax crackers of your choice. You'll need a dehydrator for this recipe, but it's oh so good.

4 red bell peppers

4–6 cloves garlic

2 teaspoons olive oil

¼ teaspoon sea salt

2 zucchini or yellow crookneck squash, peeled and chopped

¾ cup raw tahini

½ cup fresh-squeezed lemon juice

¼ cup olive oil

2½ teaspoons sea salt

1 teaspoon ground cumin

First—cut, de-vein and de-seed the peppers. Smash and peel the garlic cloves. Toss both in olive oil and ¼ teaspoon salt to thoroughly coat. Lay pieces on a Teflex sheet and tray, and dehydrate at 115 degrees for 12–24 hours. (The longer you leave in the dehydrator, the stronger and richer the flavors become.) When ready, remove from dehydrator and set aside.

In a high-speed blender or food processor, combine the remaining ingredients and blend until thick and still slightly chunky. Add in the roasted mixture and blend again until well combined and smooth.

Stacey Bradford's Nacho Dip

2 cups cashews, soaked at least 2 hours

2 small red bell peppers

1–2 jalapeños (start with a single pepper; add more to taste)

2–4 cloves garlic (2 large cloves, or 4 if small)

⅓ red onion

¼ cup lemon juice

¼ cup (heaping) nutritional yeast

¼ cup tahini

2 teaspoons salt

½ cup water (add more as needed)

Blend all ingredients until you reach the desired consistency. Serve with fresh cut veggies or flax crackers.

Sweet & Spicy Kale Chips

These are so delicious raw, but when you put the ingredients into your dehydrator for several hours, the kale becomes crispy and makes a super-tasty and healthy snack. And yes, these are kid approved!

2 bunches lacinato or dino kale (the dark, flat-leaf variety)

¼ cup olive oil

½ lemon, juiced

1 tablespoon agave nectar

1 teaspoon sea salt

A pinch of cayenne pepper

Cut kale into big pieces and place in a large bowl. Whisk together remaining ingredients and pour over kale. Work the dressing into the kale by hand; this may take a few minutes (put some love in there!). If the mixture seems too dry, you can always add a touch more oil. The kale should begin to soften and relax. You can eat this as is, or place in a dehydrator set at 115 degrees for about six hours to make chips.

Susan's Kale Chips 2.0

2 heads of curly kale, de-stemmed and cut into large pieces

¾ cup tahini (Susan makes her own tahini with a little oil and sesame seeds blended to a paste)

¼ cup Bragg Liquid Aminos

¼ cup Bragg apple cider vinegar

¼ cup water

Juice of one lemon

¼ cup nutritional yeast

1 clove garlic

Place all ingredients except kale in a food processor and run until well blended. Massage this mixture into the kale. Dry in dehydrator at 105 degrees until very crunchy.

Beggin' Strips

Believe me—you won't want to offer any of these to the dog.

1 large eggplant, thinly sliced lengthwise
½ cup olive oil
4 tablespoons umeboshi vinegar or apple cider vinegar
1 tablespoon raw honey
1 tablespoon agave nectar
1 teaspoon freshly ground black pepper

Mix together ingredients and marinate for 1 hour. Place on Teflex sheets and dehydrate for 12 hours at 105 degrees. Turn strips over and dehydrate for another 8–12 hours (without the Teflex) until crispy.

Corn Tortilla Chips

This recipe is a must-have for anyone transitioning to a high raw diet. Must have crunchy chips!

3 cups fresh corn (frozen also works fine)
1 yellow bell pepper
1 small sweet onion
2 jalapeños, seeded
2 limes, juiced
2 teaspoons cumin
2 teaspoons sea salt
1 cup golden flaxseed, ground (a bit less if using
   frozen corn)
½ cup sesame seeds (optional)

Blend all ingredients except the flax and sesame seeds in a food processor until smooth. Add the remaining ingredients and continue blending until well combined.

For the best chips, use an offset spatula to spread the dough as thinly as possible onto three 14-inch Teflex-lined dehydrator trays. Place in the dehydrator at 115 degrees for about 6 hours. Flip the sheets over and gently peel away the liners. Use a pizza cutter or knife to cut the chips and place them back into the dehydrator until crisp. This could take from 6–12 hours. Chips will keep well in an airtight container for a couple of weeks.

Susan's Onion Bread

3 large yellow onions
1 cup flaxseeds, ground in a clean coffee grinder
1 cup raw sunflower seeds, ground in a food processor
½ cup or less (to taste) Bragg Liquid Aminos or nama shoyu
¼ cup cold-pressed olive oil

Peel and halve the onions. Slice in a food processor (with slicing disc). Place onions in a large bowl and mix with the rest of the ingredients until thoroughly combined. Spread mixture over Teflex sheets until all of the mixture is used (not too thin if you want a more bread-like consistency). Dehydrate at 115 degrees for 24 hours. Flip and return to dehydrator for 12 more hours. Enjoy!

Raw Food Cleanse Entrées

Simple Stuffed Mushrooms

⅓ cup pine nuts
3 cloves garlic, minced
⅓ cup chopped cilantro leaves, packed

⅓ cup chopped basil leaves, packed
1 tablespoon fresh lemon juice
2 tablespoons Bragg Liquid Aminos, or to taste
1 cup chopped tomato
1 large container of brown button mushrooms,
   stems removed

Place all ingredients except the mushrooms and
tomato in a food processor and pulse to chop. Add
tomato and continue to pulse chop until just blended.
This mixture should be more of a pesto, not a purée.
Stuff this filling into the mushroom caps. The
mushrooms can be eaten raw or placed in a
dehydrator to warm for 2 hours at 115 degrees.

Raw Zucchini Pasta with Fresh Marinara

2 cups chopped tomatoes
1 small Vidalia onion
1 cup sun-dried tomatoes, soaked; reserve liquid
1½ tablespoons olive oil
1 clove garlic (or more if desired)
3 dates, soaked and pitted
1 sprig fresh basil
1 teaspoon sea salt
1 teaspoon red pepper flakes (optional)
2 zucchini or yellow squash
Pitted black olives

Put all ingredients in a food processor except zucchini
and olives. Blend until marinara mixture reaches the
desired consistency. Add the reserved liquid from the
sun-dried tomatoes as necessary to thin.

Use a spiral slicer, julienne peeler or vegetable
peeler to create zucchini noodles. Combine noodles

with marinara sauce and top with olives for a tasty
Italian dinner.

Sprouted Lentils with Greens and Pistachio Pesto

Sprouted lentils with greens:

2 cups sprouted lentils

1 bunch Swiss chard, steamed and chopped

5 teaspoons fresh lemon juice

1 teaspoon olive oil

¼ teaspoon maple syrup

Toss sprouted lentils, Swiss chard, lemon juice, oil and
maple syrup to coat. Place in a warm dehydrator to wilt
more quickly, if desired.

Pistachio pesto:

1 cup shelled raw pistachios

½ cup Italian parsley, tightly packed

3 tablespoons fresh lemon juice

2 teaspoons nutritional yeast (if desired)

1 tablespoon water

1 tablespoon olive oil

Blend pesto ingredients in a food processor until well
puréed. Add more water if necessary to thin.

Once lentils and chard have wilted and softened,
toss in the pesto and serve.

Mushroom Alfredo Linguine

Marinated mushrooms:

2½ cups cremini mushrooms, sliced

3 tablespoons olive oil

2 tablespoons nama shoyu

2 teaspoons apple cider vinegar

1 teaspoon raw honey

1–2 cloves garlic, minced

Toss together ingredients and marinate for 30 minutes. Drain mushrooms before using.

Alfredo sauce:

1½ cups cashews, soaked for one hour, drained

½ cup pine nuts

6 tablespoons olive oil

⅓ cup fresh lemon juice

1–2 cloves garlic, minced

1 teaspoon nutritional yeast

⅔ to 1 cup water

1–2 teaspoons sea salt

¼ cup fresh parsley, finely chopped

In a blender, blend ingredients into a smooth cream. Then fold in the parsley.

Linguine:

2 large yellow summer squash or zucchini

Using a Spirooli or standard vegetable peeler, create delicate ribbons to resemble linguine.

To serve:

Plate the linguine, cover with marinated mushrooms and top with Alfredo sauce. Garnish with chopped parsley, paprika and freshly cracked pepper.

Butternut Sage Spaghetti

These flavors go unbelievably well together. Try it—you'll like it!

Sage-pecan pesto:

1 cup fresh sage

⅔ cup raw pecans

⅓ cup olive oil (or more if needed)

1 clove garlic

1 tablespoon nutritional yeast

Spaghetti:

1 butternut squash, peeled

Olive oil, to taste

Sea salt and freshly ground black pepper, to taste

Put all ingredients for the pesto into your food processor and blend until well combined. Store pesto in an airtight container until ready to use. Spiralize or julienne-peel a butternut squash to create spaghetti noodles. Toss the noodles in a bit of olive oil, sea salt and pepper and warm in the dehydrator for about an hour, if desired, to bring out richness in flavor. Coat the spaghetti with the sage pesto mixture and serve. Garnish with a few fresh sage leaves.

Stuffed Bell Peppers

This ain't your momma's ol' stuffed bell pepper!

2 sweet red bell peppers

Cashew cheese or hummus

Diced tomatoes

Diced celery

Grated carrots

Sprouts

Fresh herbs, chopped

Cut the tops off the bell peppers. Layer the rest of the ingredients into the peppers as desired (use any amounts you like). Top with sprouts and cut herbs and place the cut tops back on for a cute presentation.

Loaded Cucumbers

Super-easy supper, great served with an avocado-based soup.

2 cucumbers
Sun & Sea Pâté (page 85)
1 bell pepper, diced
1 carrot, grated
Small handful of grated purple cabbage
Small handful of black olives, chopped

Cut the cucumbers lengthwise and remove seeds with a spoon. Fill the cucumber with pâté and then create a rainbow of color as you garnish with the remaining ingredients. Serve with flax crackers.

Spring Rolls with Peanut Sauce

For the spring rolls:
Rice paper (can be found in many grocery stores or at an Asian market)
Sprouts
Carrots, julienned
Cucumber, julienned
Fresh mint leaves
Avocado slices

For the peanut sauce:
½ cup organic peanut or almond butter
¼ cup water
1 tablespoon fresh lemon juice
2 teaspoons agave nectar
2 teaspoons nama shoyu
½ teaspoon crushed garlic
¼ teaspoon grated ginger

Dash of cayenne

Pinch of salt

To make the peanut sauce, put all ingredients in a blender and combine until creamy. To make the spring rolls, follow package directions for using rice paper. Layer ingredients in desired amounts and close up roll. (If you've never used rice paper before, you can find helpful video instructions on YouTube.)

Garden Wraps

You can put just about anything into a garden wrap, but here's my favorite version.

Red onion, finely sliced

Mushrooms, finely sliced

Baby spinach

1 tablespoon nama shoyu

1 tablespoon olive oil

Sea salt and freshly ground pepper, to taste

Crushed and minced garlic, to taste

Large-leaf collard greens, de-stemmed

Avocado, cubed

Carrot, julienned

Cucumber, julienned

Marinate the onion slices, mushrooms and spinach in a mixture of nama shoyu, olive oil, salt, pepper and garlic for at least 10 minutes to wilt. Prepare a collard leaf (lay the leaf flat to use as a wrap). Layer the onions, mushrooms, spinach, avocado, carrots and cukes and then roll up like a burrito. Slice the roll in half to serve. (A toothpick helps to keep the wrap closed when serving to a guest.)

Robin Abbott's Tomato Stacks

2 slices large ripe tomato (preferably homegrown!)
2 tablespoons Sun & Sea Pâté (page 85)
2 tablespoons Penni's Pesto (page 84)
2 tablespoons alfalfa or clover sprouts
1 teaspoon sliced black olives
Freshly ground black pepper to taste

Place one tomato slice on a plate and spread 2 tablespoons of the pâté over it. Place the second tomato slice on top, and spread with 2 tablespoons of pesto. Top with the sprouts, black olives and freshly ground pepper. Serve immediately.

Taco Salad Platter

Romaine lettuce, finely sliced
Carrots, shredded
Tomatoes, diced
Bell pepper, diced
Scallions, diced
Black olives, sliced
Black beans or kidney beans (optional)

Serve with:
Penni's Patio Salsa (page 83) and/or Cilantro Lime Dressing (page 65)
THE Best Guacamole (page 83)
Corn Tortilla Chips (page 89)

Cover a plate with shredded romaine lettuce and decorate with desired amounts of the remaining ingredients. This salad entrée is guaranteed to get your heels clicking!

Portobello Steaks
with Wilted Spinach Salad

*Even my carnivorous husband specifically requests
this dish.*

For the portobello steaks:

4 portobello mushrooms, sliced lengthwise

¾ cup olive oil

⅓ cup nama shoyu

⅓ cup apple cider vinegar

2 cloves garlic, minced

1 tablespoon fresh garden herbs of choice

½ teaspoon freshly ground black pepper

For the salad:

¼ cup olive oil

¼ cup fresh lime juice

2 teaspoons lime zest

2 small cloves garlic, minced

½ teaspoon sea salt

Freshly ground black pepper, to taste

4–5 cups fresh spinach

Final garnish:

Fresh grated nutmeg

Coat the sliced mushrooms with a marinade made
from the remaining ingredients. Allow to sit for a
couple of hours. If you have a dehydrator, warm the
marinated mushrooms at 115 degrees for at least one
hour. Make the dressing for the salad with the first six
ingredients and pour over the spinach, working the
liquid in with your hands to lightly wilt the leaves.
Arrange the dressed spinach on a plate, lay the
portobello steaks on top and serve. Grate a light

sprinkling of nutmeg over the plate for a final elegant taste.

Raw Food Cleanse Desserts

WendiLou's Berries & Cream

Fresh, seasonal berries with a sweet pumpkinseed cream sauce.

1 pint fresh raspberries
1 pint fresh blueberries

Pepita cream sauce:
1 cup raw, unsalted pumpkinseeds (pepitas)
1 cup water
2 teaspoons vanilla extract
1 tablespoon chia seeds
2 to 3 tablespoons agave nectar
Pinch of salt

Blend cream sauce ingredients in a high-speed blender or food processor until smooth. Allow the mixture to sit for 10 minutes to thicken. Add more water, if desired, to thin. Pour over a bowl full of vibrant raspberries and blueberries.

Almond Cacao Truffles

Because good people who care enough to cleanse need treats, too!

2 cups raw almonds
½ cup raw honey
¼ cup cacao nibs
Dried coconut, shredded

Process dry almonds in a food processor until you have a fairly fine meal. Transfer to a bowl, add honey and mix to create a sticky dough. Add the cacao nibs and combine well. Roll into little truffle balls and coat with shredded coconut. Keep one or two truffles in the refrigerator; the rest go in the freezer. (This will keep you out of trouble!) Truffles will keep for weeks if stored in an airtight container.

Chia Seed Ice Cream

2 tablespoons chia seeds, soaked for 15 minutes in 1 cup of
   pure water
Meat and milk of 1 Thai coconut
2 cups raw cashews, soaked for 2 hours or more
⅔ cup raw agave nectar
¼ cup coconut butter
2 tablespoons vanilla extract
Seeds of ½ vanilla bean or 2 additional teaspoons
   vanilla extract
½ teaspoon Celtic sea salt

In a high-speed blender, blend the chia gel (seeds and water) with all other ingredients until smooth. Chill in your fridge for an hour or more and then pour into your ice-cream maker, churning according to manufacturer's directions.

Delaney's Soft-serve Banana Ice Cream

I'm not a huge banana freak, but I adore spirulina and bee pollen, and frozen bananas have the perfect consistency. I rarely measure, so add however much you like of the last three ingredients. Even though I cut salt out of my diet, this really does taste better with it.

2 frozen bananas
1 tablespoon spirulina (or to taste)

1 tablespoon bee pollen (or to taste)

½ teaspoon sea salt (or to taste)

Add all ingredients to a food processor. Let it process until the mixture softens up (you may have to stop and scrape the sides). I let mine go for three minutes and then scrape. Enjoy this immediately or store in an airtight container in the freezer. Love this stuff and hope you guys do, too.

Ocean Goddess Heartland Mud "Pie"

¼ cup flaxseeds, ground

⅓ cup sunflower seeds, ground briefly so there are still a few chunks of seeds

1 tablespoon (or less) raw cacao powder

1 teaspoon Dandy Blend coffee substitute (not necessary, but I like the coffee flavor)

Splash of coconut milk (or any nut milk, or rice or soy in a pinch—or, heck, even water!)

Agave nectar or honey, to taste

Mix it all up, in the order listed. Add enough liquid to make the consistency "muddy" and then add sweetener to taste.

Susan's Delicious Raw Carrot Cake

A great dessert to make when entertaining or going to a party. Just don't keep this around your house to tempt you!

Cake:

¼ cup fresh moist dates, pitted

¾ cup shredded/grated carrot

3 tablespoons flax meal

¼ cup dried unsweetened coconut

1 teaspoon vanilla

2 tablespoons agave nectar

¼ tablespoon cinnamon

¼ teaspoon sea salt

⅛ teaspoon nutmeg

⅛ teaspoon ground ginger

½ cup chopped nuts (pecans or walnuts)

¼ cup raisins

Blend dates until they are a paste and then add everything else except the nuts, raisins and about a handful of the carrot shavings. Continue blending until ingredients are well combined, then add nuts, raisins and the rest of the carrot shavings and pulse just until blended. Mold this mixture into the desired shape and place in a dehydrator for about 4 hours at 115 degrees or until firm enough to hold frosting.

Frosting:

1 cup cashews (soaked in water for 2 hours)

¼ cup agave nectar

2 tablespoons fresh orange juice

2 tablespoons coconut oil

½ to 1 teaspoon vanilla

Pinch of Celtic sea salt

Place all frosting ingredients in a blender and process until smooth and creamy. Refrigerate frosting to thicken if necessary. Frost cake and sprinkle some decorative carrot shavings on top to serve.

Section II—Maintaining Your Cleanse for Life

Delicious and nutritious recipes for maintaining a toxin-free body for life.

Lifestyle Juices

Juicy Pink

Although grapefruit juice is touted for its ability to lower cholesterol, avoid it if you are taking certain medications or undergoing chemotherapy. Check with your health care provider if you have concerns.

2 pink grapefruits, peeled and seeded
2 soft ripe pears, cored
½ inch fresh ginger

Push all ingredients through a juicer. Serve over ice and decorate with thin slices of pear and grapefruit.

Tangy Green Tease

2 kiwis, peeled
1 cup green grapes
¼ ripe honeydew melon, peeled

Push all ingredients through your juicer.

Citrus Blast

I've been taught that this is the juice to drink when you want to reduce cellulite and fat deposits.

3 oranges
3 grapefruits
1 lemon

Juice the citrus fruits using a citrus press, a blender or a juicer.

Simple Pleasure

This combination is super-cleansing, and because of its good blend of sodium and potassium it is a very balancing drink.

2 cups fresh spinach
5 stalks celery
3 crisp ripe apples

Push all ingredients through a juicer. Drink immediately for best results.

Clear & Calm

This mild yet flavorful juice is a favorite. The beta-carotene of the melon is excellent for vision; add the calming qualities of romaine and you have a winning combination.

½ head romaine lettuce
½ medium cantaloupe, peeled

Push ingredients through a juicer and serve over ice for a refreshing drink.

Anemia Buster

Regular consumption of this iron-rich combination will help keep anemia at bay. Iron is essential for carrying oxygen in the bloodstream, and this uniquely delicious juice will energize and revitalize even the most sluggish of systems.

3 ripe apricots
3 carrots

Handful of spinach
½ lemon, peeled
2 teaspoons kelp powder
1 tablespoon ground pumpkinseeds

Juice the first four ingredients, then transfer to a
blender and add the kelp powder and ground
pumpkinseeds. Blend, then drink immediately to
invigorate and energize.

Clean Sweep

*Time to clean house? This vitamin- and mineral-
rich juice is chock-full of sweet goodness. Drink
this whenever you feel like giving your system a
thorough cleansing.*

Handful of green grapes
Several sprigs fresh parsley
3 carrots
2 stalks celery

Push the grapes and parsley through the juicer,
followed by the carrots and celery.

Pure Vitality

*This vibrant blend is guaranteed to get your taste
buds tingling.*

1 medium beet
6 carrots
1 organic lemon
1-inch piece of fresh ginger

Feed all ingredients through a juicer, including the
peel of the lemon. Enjoy!

Liquid Sunshine

The high glycemic index of carrots and tangerines is nicely balanced by the addition of golden flaxseeds. This is a perfect morning drink and a great way to get plenty of vitamin C, beta-carotene, omega-3 fatty acid and fiber.

6 carrots
4 tangerines (or oranges), peeled
2 teaspoons golden flaxseeds, ground
½ teaspoon orange zest

Run the carrots and tangerines through a juicer. Mix in the ground flax and orange zest for a brilliant wake-up for your taste buds.

I Can See Now

Carrots and pears blend well together. The alfalfa sprouts add a punch of vitamins A, C and K, while also balancing the glycemic index of the juice.

6 carrots
4 pears
2 cups alfalfa sprouts

Run everything through a juicer. Garnish with a carrot curl and a few sprouts.

Sweet Basil

Basil adds a unique flavor infusion to this delicious, beautifying juice. It's a perfect substitute for an evening cocktail because of the relaxing effect produced by the basil.

½ cup fresh basil
8 apples

6 stalks celery

1 large cucumber

Push basil through the juicer first, followed by the other fruits and vegetables, for the greatest efficiency.

Sassy Bunny

I named this titillating combination after a friend of mine whose online screen name is Sassy Bunny. Although I won't recommend it here, Ms. Bunny would likely prefer this juice with an ounce or two of organic vodka.

6 carrots

3 Gala or other ripe apples

1 organic lemon, peeled

1-inch piece fresh ginger

Freshly grated lemon zest, for garnish

Juice the first four ingredients, leaving the lemon zest for the final garnish.

Lifestyle Smoothies & Shakes

Protein Purifier

8 leaves romaine lettuce

1 cup grapes

1 medium orange, peeled

¼ cup hemp nuts

1 cup water

1 cup crushed ice

Combine all ingredients in a blender until smooth and creamy.

Get Your Green On

1 banana, fresh or frozen

1 cup strawberries

2–3 handfuls of spinach

Fresh orange juice, to taste (use water if you have high
   blood sugar)

Blend ingredients well and enjoy!

Orange-ango

1 mango

2 tangerines

¼ teaspoon vanilla powder

½ cup orange juice

Combine ingredients in a blender until creamy.

Basic Black

3 cups black grapes

2 cups fresh blackberries

2 cups frozen cherries

Place all ingredients in a high-speed blender and run
until smooth. You may prefer to strain the seeds before
drinking, but it isn't necessary.

Supermodel Blend

*This is an updated version of one of my recipes that
was featured in* The Raw 50 *by Carol Alt.*

1 frozen banana

1 cup frozen strawberries

½ cup fresh almond milk

1 large orange, juiced

1 tablespoon raw honey
2 teaspoons Crystal Manna Flakes

Combine all ingredients in a blender, mixing until smooth. Now go get out on the catwalk!

Warrior Blend

Hardcore superhero fuel!

1 banana
2 or more cups frozen berries of choice
Handful of soaked raw pumpkin and sunflower seeds
1 tablespoon raw almond or cashew butter
1 tablespoon flaxseed oil
1 tablespoon super green food powder, of your choice
½ serving of vanilla Sun Warrior Protein
1 tablespoon maca powder
1 tablespoon ground golden flaxseeds
Fresh organic apple juice, enough to liquefy mixture

Place all ingredients in a high-speed blender and whip into creamy perfection.

Penni-colada

1 orange, peeled
½ cup pineapple, fresh or frozen
1 frozen banana
½ cup almond milk
A splash of vanilla extract

Place everything in a blender and combine until smooth and creamy.

Dreamsicle Shake

1 young Thai coconut, milk and meat

2 frozen bananas

3 dates

Juice of a ripe navel orange (just hand-squeeze the orange
straight into the blender)

1 tablespoon honey

1 teaspoon vanilla

Ice cubes

Place all ingredients, except ice, in blender and blend
till smooth. Add ice cubes gradually until desired
consistency is reached.

Bradbury's Tropical Smoothie

4 fresh peaches

¼ fresh pineapple

1 mango, peeled and pitted

6–8 large strawberries

2–3 cups fresh almond milk

Whiz together in Vita-Mix. Enjoy!

Blue Moon

1 cup frozen blueberries

1 cup frozen peaches

3 cups fresh apple juice

1 teaspoon fresh grated ginger

¼ teaspoon fresh grated nutmeg

Raw honey to taste

Place all ingredients into the blender and mix
until smooth.

Egg-free "Egg Nog" Smoothie

I'm one of those odd people who never liked the smell or taste of egg nog. Something about it reminds me of glue. This raw vegan egg nog is so delicious, I don't even know why they keep making the traditional version.

3 cups almond milk
5 large dates, pitted and soaked
2 very ripe bananas (I prefer mine frozen)
1 teaspoon raw vanilla powder
⅛ teaspoon cinnamon
⅛ teaspoon nutmeg

Place all ingredients in a high-speed blender and combine until smooth and creamy. Sift a bit of freshly grated nutmeg on top to finish.

Digestive Healer

1 young Thai coconut, meat and water
1 cup frozen papaya
1 frozen banana
6 collard leaves, de-veined
1 cup vanilla hemp milk
1 package stevia or 1 tablespoon agave nectar
Crushed ice

Blend together all ingredients until smooth.

Peaches & Crème

Simple and delicious, this recipe is at its best when fresh local peaches are in season. If using fresh peaches, simply add crushed ice to your blender.

1 small bag frozen organic peaches
2 cups macadamia or almond milk
½ teaspoon vanilla powder
2 tablespoons raw honey

Put all ingredients into a high-speed blender and combine until well blended.

Cacao Banana

The combo of chocolate and banana has always appealed to me—it'll keep you sustained for hours.

1 cup Brazil nut milk
1 tablespoon raw cacao powder
1 tablespoon almond butter
1 teaspoon maca powder
1 teaspoon vanilla extract

Place all ingredients in your blender and blend until smooth. Yummy!

Lifestyle Smart Cocktails

Melon Kiwi-tini

A kiwi has as much vitamin C as an orange and 10 percent of the RDA of vitamin E, with only 50 calories per kiwi.

2 kiwis, peeled
½ ripe honeydew melon, peeled
2 tablespoons blue agave nectar
2 tablespoons fresh-squeezed lime juice
½ cup kombucha
Extra kiwi slices and 2 sprigs mint, for garnish

Chop the fruit and place in a blender with the lime juice and agave nectar; blend on high until smooth and puréed. Add more agave nectar to taste, throw in a handful of ice and blend again on high. Pour into 2 large martini glasses, top with kombucha and garnish with thin slices of peeled kiwi and mint. Serves 2.

Blood Orange Raw Mojito

Juice of two blood oranges
Juice of two limes
1 bunch muddled fresh mint
A good squeeze of agave nectar
2 cups (16 ounces) Rejuvelac or kombucha

Place all ingredients in a martini shaker and gently mix. Pour into chilled martini or wine glasses; garnish with a sprig of fresh mint. Savor and allow the tensions of the day to fall away.

Mint Julep

1 cup fresh mint leaves, plus extra sprigs for garnish
2 cups fresh pineapple juice (the juice of one small pineapple)
Juice of 2 lemons
1+ tablespoon raw honey or agave nectar (if you are feeling edgy)
1 teaspoon lemon zest
A good splash of GT's Organic Raw Kombucha (Original flavor), club soda or sparkling water

Juice mint, pineapple and lemons in your juicer. Add honey or agave nectar and lemon zest and let sit in your refrigerator for 30 minutes or more. Before serving, add kombucha, sparkling water, or club soda and pour over ice. Garnish with mint sprigs.

Fuzzy Navel

1 cup pecans, soaked and drained
2 oranges, zest and segments
½ cup soaked dates, pitted
1 teaspoon vanilla powder or vanilla extract

Place pecans in a blender with 2 cups pure water. Blend into a thick, rich milk, straining if a smooth consistency is desired. Add orange zest, orange segments, soaked dates and vanilla. Continue blending until well combined. Serve in pretty glasses with an orange slice on the rim for garnish.

Kumquat Caipiroska

The caipirinha is Brazil's national cocktail that is made with cachaça, Brazil's most common distilled alcoholic beverage. A Caipiroska is made like the caipirinha, but vodka is used instead. A wide variety of fresh fruits can easily be used in place of lime.

2 limes, cut into wedges
2 tablespoons agave nectar
Pint of kumquats (12 ounces), halved and juiced by hand
¼ cup kombucha (or go ahead and live a little . . . organic
  vodka is widely available)

Place lime slices and agave nectar into a large cocktail shaker or pitcher, and muddle (mash the two ingredients together using a muddler or a wooden spoon). Pour in the kumquat juice and kombucha/vodka, and gently mix or shake until combined. Serve over crushed ice in a chilled martini glass or tall glass. Add a slice of lime and mint-leaf garnish on the rim of your glass for a perfect presentation.

Chocotini

*This non-alcoholic lift is nutritious and delicious cold,
or it can be heated to make a comforting hot
chocolate for winter nights by the fire.*

½ cup hazelnuts, soaked
2 tablespoons cacao powder
2 tablespoons agave nectar (I use less)
½ teaspoon raw vanilla powder or 1 teaspoon
   vanilla extract
1 tablespoon grated cacao butter
Pinch of salt
1 ounce organic vodka (optional)
1 tablespoon small raw cacao nibs, for garnish

In a high-speed blender, mix the soaked hazelnuts and
1 cup water until smooth, then strain to make a thick,
milky cream. You can add a bit more water if it's too
thick. Add the cacao powder, agave nectar, vanilla,
cacao butter, salt and vodka (if using), and blend again
until well incorporated.

Serving options: Pour into a cocktail shaker, shake
with ice, and serve in a martini glass with nibs for
garnish. Or gently heat in a saucepan on low until
nicely warmed.

Spiced (Not Spiked) Holiday Punch

*Great served in a punch bowl at the holidays! This
recipe will serve 6 guests, but can easily be doubled or
tripled for larger crowds.*

6 apples
8 oranges, peeled
1 lemon, peeled
1 cup fresh cranberries

½ cup agave nectar

¼ teaspoon cinnamon

¼ teaspoon five-spice powder

1-liter bottle sparkling mineral water

Slices of citrus and a handful of frozen cranberries
  for garnish

Juice the apples, oranges, lemon and cranberries and
then pour into a blender. Add the agave nectar and
spices and blend until thoroughly mixed. Serve in
festive glasses with a ratio of ⅔ punch to ⅓ sparkling
mineral water and finish with sliced fruit and a few
cranberries floating on top.

Apple Rosemary Infusion

1 large sprig of rosemary, plus another small sprig
  for garnish

10 apples, juiced

Place large rosemary sprig in a small saucepan with
½ cup hot water, then cover the pan and allow the
mixture to infuse for a minute or two. Strain the
rosemary water, discard sprig and blend the infused
water with the freshly squeezed apple juice. Serve over
ice with a small sprig of fresh rosemary in the glass.

Lifestyle Dressings & Sauces

The Mother Sauce

*This dressing can be used for many purposes. I try to
always keep some on hand in an airtight container in
the refrigerator.*

1 cup cashews or macadamia nuts, soaked and drained

2 tablespoons fresh lemon or lime juice

1 tablespoon raw honey
1 tablespoon dried onion flakes
1 teaspoon fresh basil
1 teaspoon fresh cut herbs of choice
2 cloves garlic
¼ teaspoon sea salt
Pinch cayenne pepper

Put the soaked, drained nuts into a high-speed blender, adding 1 cup of pure water to blend well. Add the remaining ingredients and combine until creamy.

Raw Ketchup

For a smoky, southwestern twist, try adding one soaked chipotle pepper to the ketchup.

2 tomatoes, chopped
1 cup sun-dried tomatoes
Juice of ½ lemon
1 pitted date
Sea salt and freshly ground black pepper, to taste

Combine these ingredients in a high-speed blender, blending until smooth and well combined.

Honey Lime Vinaigrette

I could eat this dressing on everything, every day. That's how much I love it.

½ cup olive oil
1/3 cup raw local honey
¼ cup fresh lime juice
½ teaspoon lime zest
1/8 teaspoon freshly ground nutmeg
Sea salt and freshly cracked black pepper to taste

Whisk all ingredients to emulsify. This dressing will keep well in an airtight jar in the refrigerator for at least 2 weeks.

Lifestyle Hearty Breakfast

Ruby's Raw Cherry Granola

2 apples, any variety

1 generous cup dates, soaked (drain and reserve water)

½ cup maple syrup

½ cup fresh orange juice

1 tablespoon orange zest

2 teaspoons cinnamon

2 teaspoons sea salt

½ cup walnuts, soaked a couple of hours

3 cups pecans, soaked

2 cups almonds, soaked

2 cups buckwheat, rinsed well and soaked a few hours

3 cups thick rolled oats (optional since they're not technically raw)

1 cup golden flaxseeds, ground or whole

1 cup dried cherries

1 cup pumpkinseeds (optional)

1 cup goji berries (optional)

1 tablespoon vanilla extract

Start by adding the following ingredients to your food processor: one apple, dates and about ¼ cup of the soak water, maple syrup, orange juice, zest, cinnamon, salt and walnuts. Grind until completely smooth, then transfer to a large mixing bowl.

Dice the remaining apple and add it to the mixing bowl. Place the pecans and almonds in the food processor and coarsely chop nuts in a few quick pulses.

Add them to the bowl along with the apple mixture. Then add all remaining ingredients to the bowl and combine well.

Spread the granola on lined dehydrator trays and dehydrate at 115 degrees for 6–8 hours. Peel off the Teflex sheeting and continue to dehydrate until the granola is crunchy. Break into pieces and, once completely cooled, store in airtight containers. This recipe makes a huge supply that will last you for months. It's fun to make this with a friend (one who has a big nine-tray dehydrator!) and share the love.

Raw Morning Power Bars

1 cup nuts of choice
1 cup medjool or other soft dates
1 teaspoon lemon juice
Pinch of salt

In the food processor, blend nuts until they form a mealy texture. Don't blend to a powder; the bars taste better with tiny pieces of nuts in them. Next, press the dates to a paste. I do this by hand in a little bowl. If you do it in your blender or food processor, the dates will stick to the blade, so hand chopping may be easier. When a paste has formed, add the nut meal, lemon juice and salt and mix by hand into dough.

Make two long ropes from the dough by rolling it over your cutting board. Make the top and edges flat by pressing with a flat wooden spoon. Cut each rope into three pieces.

Wrap your individual bars in plastic and store them in the refrigerator. This will keep your bars firm so they will travel better, if necessary.

Katie's Blueberry Crumble

1 vanilla bean, opened and scraped

¼ cup walnuts

¼ cup oats

1 tablespoon honey

1 date, pitted and chopped

1 teaspoon extra virgin coconut oil (optional, but it is tasty)

Add vanilla-bean scrapings and walnuts to a food processor, grinding until medium coarse. Add oats and honey and blend till sticky and mixed (oats should now be tiny slivers in the mix). Add date pieces gradually and grind till well mixed. Transfer mixture to bowl and press flat. Spread 1 teaspoon of coconut oil on top. After evenly coated, break up the crust into small crumbs with a spoon and chill crumbs in the icebox for a few minutes.

I can eat this all by myself. It makes a serving or two. I sprinkle the crumbs on top of a cup of frozen blueberries that have thawed slightly. I bet this mixture would make a great pie crust, too.

Manna Bread Layered Breakfast Toast

Although manna bread is not technically raw, it's a wonderfully nutritious sprouted-grain bread that has been cooked at a very low temperature, therefore retaining essential nutrients. This is a decadent but healthy recipe for any time of day.

For the vanilla crème sauce:

1½ cups cashews, soaked for a few hours or overnight, drained

3 tablespoons agave nectar

2 teaspoons vanilla extract

½ vanilla bean, scraped

Blend all ingredients in your blender, adding pure water as needed to achieve a thick but creamy consistency. Sauce will keep in your refrigerator for three days if stored in a glass container, with plastic wrap pressed against the surface of the sauce to create an airtight seal.

For assembly:

1 loaf manna bread, thawed

Raw almond butter, or other nut butter

1 banana, sliced

Fresh seasonal berries

Slice manna bread into ⅓-inch-thick slices. You can either toast the bread or eat as is. On each slice, spread a thin layer of almond butter first and then add a thin layer of banana slices. Next, add the vanilla crème sauce, and top with berries.

Lifestyle Soups

Strawberry Cloud

This is a chilled summer fruit soup, but can also be enjoyed as a smoothie.

1 Thai coconut, meat and milk

1 pint fresh strawberries

5 oranges, peeled

1 tablespoon raw honey

½ teaspoon raw vanilla powder

1 cup crushed ice

Crack open a Thai coconut, pouring out and reserving the water and extracting the meat. Place into a high-speed blender along with the strawberries, oranges, honey, vanilla and crushed ice. Blend together until smooth and creamy. Serve chilled.

Ruby's Smokin' Hot Tomato Soup

2 cups fresh tomatoes (I like cherry or grape baby ones)
2 cups sun-dried tomatoes, soaked (save the soak water, about 1+ cup)
½ cup olive oil
½ cup raw cashews, soaked for 1–2 hours
1 clove garlic
¼ cup shallot, chopped
1 tablespoon red pepper flakes
1 tablespoon agave nectar or raw honey
1 teaspoon smoked sea salt (if you have it; otherwise substitute regular sea salt)
Fresh herbs for garnish

Blend all ingredients, including soak water from the sun-dried tomatoes, in your blender. Combine until the mixture reaches a creamy consistency. Add pure water to thin as needed. If you want to reduce the heat, use fewer red pepper flakes.

Nectar of the Mexican Goddesses

When my whole neighborhood celebrated Cinco de Mayo with Mexican food and margaritas, I decided I didn't want to miss out on the fun and festivities. This creamy, delicious blended soup was just the thing to put me in the mood for a celebration!

2 ears of organic corn, kernels cut from the ear
2 stalks celery
½ red bell pepper

1 small yellow onion
¼ bunch fresh cilantro
Juice of 1–2 limes
1 jalapeño
Dash of ground cayenne pepper
Sprinkling of mace or nutmeg
Celtic sea salt to taste

Place all ingredients in a high-powered blender and combine until smooth and creamy.

Indian Curry Silk

4 stalks celery
2 stalks lemongrass
3 carrots
2 jalapeños
1 small red bell pepper
3 scallions
1 small knob of ginger
½ cup fresh basil
1 large handful of cilantro
2 limes, peeled
1 young coconut, water
1 tablespoon avocado oil
½ teaspoon Indian curry
Raw honey to taste

Push the first 10 ingredients through your juicer, then transfer the juice to your Vita-Mix and add the young coconut water, avocado oil, curry, and honey. Blend for about 20 seconds, and enjoy!

Cream of Asparagus Soup

½ cup soaked cashews

2 cups Balancing Broth (page 76)

2 stalks celery

1 clove garlic

½ teaspoon fresh thyme

1 bunch asparagus

Put all ingredients into a high-speed blender and combine until smooth and creamy. Garnish with asparagus tips and fresh chopped herbs.

Minestrone

3 cups Balancing Broth (page 76)

3 cups diced fresh tomatoes

1 cup chopped onion

1 cup shredded cabbage

½ cup chopped carrots

½ cup chopped celery

1 tablespoon fresh basil

1 clove garlic, minced

2 cups cooked white beans

1 medium zucchini, sliced ¼-inch thick and halved

2 tablespoons grated Parmigiano-Reggiano for
  topping (optional)

In a large stock pot, mix broth, tomatoes, onion, cabbage, carrots, celery, basil and garlic. Bring to a boil, reduce heat, cover and simmer for 20 minutes. Add water if necessary. Stir in beans and zucchini, return to boiling, reduce heat, cover and simmer for an additional 10 minutes. Serve in bowls and top with freshly grated raw cheese, if desired.

Lifestyle Side Dishes, Salads & Snacks

Pesto Italiano

*This unconventional pesto is delicious over pasta,
stuffed into mushrooms or served with an assortment
of raw crackers and sliced Roma tomatoes.*

1 cup raw almonds
½ cup fresh Italian parsley
1–2 cloves garlic
⅓ cup green olives (black can be substituted)
¼ teaspoon crushed red pepper flakes
¾ cup olive oil
Sea salt and freshly cracked black pepper to taste

Place all ingredients into a food processor and pulse
until finely chopped, adding a bit of water if necessary
to achieve the right consistency.

Quinoa Tabbouleh with Pistachios

*True Middle Eastern tabbouleh is more about the mint
and herbs than the grain that is used. This dish can be
made 100 percent raw with sprouted quinoa. It's
wonderful served inside a lettuce leaf for a filling
entrée. This salad becomes even better on the second
day, so make plenty!*

3 tablespoons olive oil
¼ cup fresh lemon juice
1 clove garlic, minced
Sea salt and freshly ground black pepper to taste
½ cup quinoa, cooked (or substitute sprouted quinoa for a
   100 percent raw recipe)
1½ cups pistachio nuts, finely chopped
1 small cucumber, finely chopped

½ cup finely chopped fresh tomato

5 green onions, finely chopped

⅓ cup chopped fresh mint (add more if you like mint)

Whisk oil, lemon juice and garlic together in a bowl, and season with salt and pepper. Set aside. Bring 1 cup water to a boil in a medium saucepan. Add quinoa; cover, reduce heat to low and cook until the water is absorbed, about 13 minutes. Transfer to a large bowl and let cool.

Add pistachios, cucumber, tomato, onions and mint to the quinoa, then pour in the dressing and toss well to coat.

White Bean Dip

This tangy, Greek-style bean dip is best served with an assortment of fresh veggies. It is a crowd-pleaser! It's also a great addition to a healthy lettuce or sprouted-grain veggie wrap.

2 cups cooked cannellini or Great Northern beans

2 cloves garlic, minced

2 tablespoons fresh lemon juice

2 tablespoons olive oil

¼ teaspoon sea salt

⅛ teaspoon freshly cracked black pepper

2 teaspoons fresh chopped herbs (oregano, basil, etc.)

Combine all ingredients in a food processor and blend until smooth. Chill for a few hours to allow the flavors to blend and intensify.

Penni's Picnic Potato Salad

8 Yukon Gold or 4 sweet potatoes, skin on

½ cup chopped red, yellow or orange bell pepper

2 cups chopped celery
½ cup minced red onion
2 tablespoons chopped fresh parsley
The Mother Sauce, to taste (page 116)

Scrub and cube potatoes. Boil, drain and cool. Add
in all other ingredients, and toss in The Mother Sauce
to dress.

Wild Rice Salad

*This dish can be adjusted to 100 percent raw by using
sprouted quinoa instead of cooked wild rice.*

For the salad:
2 cups cooked wild rice
½ cup shredded carrot
½ cup shredded zucchini
½ cup minced red bell pepper
½ cup shredded celery
½ cup shredded purple cabbage

For the dressing:
¼ cup mellow white miso
¼ cup raw honey
¼ tablespoon apple cider vinegar
2 tablespoons olive oil
2 tablespoons fresh orange juice
1 tablespoon fresh parsley
1 tablespoon fresh basil
Sea salt to taste

Combine all ingredients for the salad in a large bowl.
Set aside. Put all the dressing ingredients into a
blender and blend until well emulsified. Then pour
the dressing over the salad and mix well. This salad

will keep for several days if refrigerated in an airtight container.

Marvelous Marinated Bean Salad

2 cups cooked garbanzo beans, cooled
1 cup cooked black beans, cooled
1 cup cooked red kidney beans, cooled
1 medium onion, chopped
½ cup chopped orange or red bell pepper
¼ cup apple cider vinegar
¼ cup fresh lime juice
½ cup olive oil
2 tablespoons agave nectar
1 jalapeño, minced
1 clove garlic, minced

Combine beans, onion and bell pepper in a large mixing bowl. Put the rest of the ingredients in a blender and blend until emulsified. Pour the dressing over the bean mixture, coating well. Place in an airtight container in the refrigerator until ready to serve.

Cheesy Broccoli & Cauliflower

2 bunches of broccoli
½ head cauliflower
¼ cup finely sliced red onion
⅓ cup tahini
¼ cup lime juice
½ cup sunflower seeds
¼ cup sesame seeds, plus a bit more for garnish
2 cloves garlic
2 teaspoons nutritional yeast
Celtic sea salt to taste

Chop broccoli and cauliflower into small, bite-size pieces, then place in a large bowl with the sliced red onion. Combine the remaining ingredients in a high-speed blender, blend until smooth, and add to the broccoli/cauliflower/onion mixture. Mix well and garnish with sesame seeds.

Lifestyle Entrées

Pasta with Leeks, Radicchio, Walnut Pesto & Parmesan

This is a crisp and deliciously fresh meal. Many high-quality Parmigiano-Reggiano cheeses are made with raw milk. Check with your cheesemonger, or simply omit this ingredient for a raw, vegan meal.

4 cups thinly sliced leeks (include some of the dark green part)
4 tablespoons olive oil, divided
½ cup fresh Italian parsley, plus extra for garnish
¼ cup walnuts, plus extra for garnish
2 teaspoons lemon juice
1 clove garlic
Sea salt and freshly cracked black pepper to taste
1 large zucchini, processed through a spiral slicer for pasta
2 cups thinly sliced radicchio
Parmigiano-Reggiano, thinly shaved (optional)

Toss leeks with just enough olive oil to coat. Place in a warm dehydrator for at least an hour. Purée parsley, walnuts, lemon juice, garlic and the remainder of the olive oil in a mini-prep or food processor until a coarse purée forms. Season with sea salt and freshly cracked pepper to taste. Toss this pesto with the zucchini noodles, the leek mixture and the radicchio. Garnish

with additional walnuts, fresh parsley and shaved
Parmesan cheese.

Homemade Chili-in-the-Raw

*This recipe was created one evening when I decided to
hold a meaty-cooked vs. vegan-raw chili smackdown
with my husband. This recipe went into the "keeper"
file that very night!*

For the "meaty" base:

1 cup soaked almonds or walnuts, chopped well in a food
   processor

1 cup carrots, chopped well in a food processor

1 medium portobello mushroom or 5 shiitake
   mushrooms, chopped

½ cup minced celery

½ medium red onion, minced

½ medium red bell pepper, chopped

1 jalapeño pepper, finely minced

½ cup black olives, chopped (optional)

For the rich chili sauce:

1 cup sun-dried tomatoes, soaked (retain 1 cup of
   soak water)

1 cup chopped fresh tomatoes

1 tablespoon raw honey or ¼ cup raisins

1 tablespoon olive oil

1 tablespoon minced fresh leeks, or other mild/sweet onion

2 cloves garlic

2 tablespoons fresh oregano

2 tablespoons chili powder

1 teaspoon cumin

2 teaspoons apple cider vinegar

1–2 teaspoons Celtic sea salt (only 1 teaspoon if you
   included olives in the base)

For the topping:
Chopped cilantro, chopped black olives, minced red onion, fresh avocado chunks

Combine the processed almonds and carrots in a large bowl. Add the rest of the ingredients for the chili base, and toss to mix. Set aside. Place all ingredients for the chili sauce in a high-speed blender and process until well combined and creamy. (You can add water as necessary to thin the sauce.) Pour the sauce over the base and stir to blend. Warm in a dehydrator for 1–2 hours if desired.

Top with chopped cilantro, minced red onion, chopped black olives and/or fresh avocado chunks. Chili will keep well in an airtight container for 3–5 days in your refrigerator.

Black Beans & Rice

This is a satisfying, nutritious and hearty dish for a cold winter night.

¾ cup Balancing Broth (page 76)
1 medium onion, chopped
4 cloves garlic, minced
2 cups cooked black beans, drained
2 cups diced fresh tomatoes
¼ teaspoon chili powder
2 cups cooked long-grain brown rice

In a saucepan, cook the onion and garlic in a couple of tablespoons of Balancing Broth until tender. Stir in beans, tomatoes, remaining broth and chili powder. Bring to a boil, then reduce heat and simmer for about 15 minutes. Add the rice, stirring well to combine, and serve.

Hipped-Up Sweet Potato Cashew Casserole

My mother used to make something like this, but it involved lots of butter, brown sugar and marshmallows. I like this version much better, and I can serve it to holiday guests without any guilt or shame.

6 medium sweet potatoes
2 cups chopped fresh peaches (frozen organic peaches are also fine)
⅓ cup agave nectar or maple syrup
½ teaspoon ground fresh ginger
2 tablespoons coconut oil
¼ cup cashews, coarsely chopped

Scrub potatoes and cut into ½-inch slices. In a 2-quart rectangular baking dish, make a layer using half the potatoes and half the peaches. In a bowl, combine the agave nectar, coconut oil and ginger. Use half of this mixture to glaze the potatoes and peaches in the baking dish. Then repeat the layering with the remaining half of the potatoes and peaches, and spread the rest of the glaze on top. Bake, covered, at 350 degrees for 45 minutes, stirring once. Remove from oven and sprinkle with cashews. Bake an additional 15 minutes, uncovered, until the potatoes are tender. Serves 6.

Andrea's Awesome E.A.T. Sandwich

One of the superstars of Raw Food Rehab, Andrea, put together this amazing raw sandwich to live for. Think BLT, only way better.

Onion bread
The Mother Sauce (page 116)

Eggplant bacon (see Beggin' Strips recipe, page 89)

Sliced tomatoes

Green leaf lettuce

Sprouts

Avocado slices or guacamole

Take a slice of onion bread and spread with a layer of The Mother Sauce. Begin layering the sandwich with lettuce, tomato and eggplant, finishing it off with a generous layer of guacamole or sliced avocado and sprouts. Cover with a second piece of onion bread.

Portobello Burgers by Amie Sue

For the veggie burgers:

1 cup cremini or brown button mushrooms

1 cup pecans

Handful of cilantro

1½ cups carrots

½ cup dried tomatoes

1 teaspoon cumin

1 teaspoon coriander

½ teaspoon sea salt

½ teaspoon ground chili powder

Few squirts of olive oil

Freshly cracked black pepper

For the buns:

4 portobello mushrooms

¼ cup olive oil

¼ cup Bragg Liquid Aminos

Mix all of the burger ingredients in a food processor, adding a bit of water to help combine. Shape the mix into patties and place on mesh trays in your dehydrator. (This recipe makes about two patties, but you may end up with additional patties that will keep well in the refrigerator for several days.) Dehydrate patties for 6 hours, then turn over and dehydrate another 6 hours.

After the patties have been in the dehydrator for about two and a half hours, begin preparing the portobello buns. Cut the stems from the portobello mushrooms and gently scoop some of the center out so that the burgers will fit between the mushrooms. Brush the inside and outside of the mushrooms with the combined olive oil and Bragg's. Place the prepared buns into the dehydrator after the patties have been in for about 3 hours.

Once the buns and patties are as firm and dry as you like them, remove them from the dehydrator and build your burger. In addition to the usual lettuce-and-tomato garnish, I recommend avocado slices, Bubbies raw pickles, sliced sweet onion, The Mother Sauce (page 116), Raw Ketchup (page 117) and Raw Mustard (page 67).

Gracious Grain with Voluptuous Veggies

A very easy cold-weather entrée is simply prepared whole grains served with steamed root vegetables.

Pair 1 cup cooked grain (amaranth, buckwheat, millet, quinoa, brown or wild rice) with a combination of any of the following:

Carrots
Celery
Onion
Broccoli
Cauliflower
Bell pepper

Green beans
Squash
Mushrooms

Once you've cooked the grain and steamed the veggies, use your choice of Bragg Liquid Aminos or a bit of nama shoyu to add flavor. Garnish with fresh herbs if available.

Stuffed Baked Potato Supper

Another hearty vegan dinner for those colder months or for those still transitioning to a raw-foods diet. When choosing potatoes for baking, always select organic.

For the vegetable stuffing
  (any combination of the following):
Garlic, minced
Onions, coarsely chopped
Bell peppers, chopped
Broccoli, chopped
Mushrooms, sliced

To prepare:
1 baked potato
1 tablespoon coconut oil (plus a bit more for topping,
  if desired)
½ cup white wine (can omit and use only Balancing Broth)
Balancing Broth (page 76)
Fresh herbs
Sea salt and freshly cracked black pepper to taste
Fresh salsa

In a stainless steel skillet, heat coconut oil, then add onion and garlic (in desired amounts), sautéing until soft. Add white wine and the additional vegetables.

Add Balancing Broth as necessary to finish cooking; veggies should be tender, yet not overcooked. Season with fresh herbs, sea salt and pepper.

Cut open the baked potato and fill with the sautéed vegetables. Add a touch of coconut oil and/or fresh salsa if desired.

Lifestyle Desserts

Seasonal Fruit Crisp

Any seasonal fruit will work in this versatile recipe. I just happened to use peaches and my family raved over it.

½ cup almonds

½ cup pecans

½ cup macadamia nuts (next time I'll used sprouted oats)

1–2 tablespoons coconut butter

½ cup shredded coconut

½ teaspoon cinnamon

½ teaspoon nutmeg or pumpkin pie spice

¼ teaspoon sea salt

6–8 ripe peaches, peeled and sliced (or substitute other fresh fruit)

1 tablespoon lemon juice

½ cup maple syrup

Put the nuts into a food processor and pulse until well crumbled. Add in coconut butter; pulse. Transfer ingredients to a large bowl and fold in shredded coconut, cinnamon, nutmeg and salt.

In another bowl, combine peach slices, lemon juice and maple syrup, coating the peaches well. Pour peach mixture into a square glass baking dish. Next, cover the peach layer completely with the crumble mixture. Warm in a dehydrator for a couple of hours before serving, if desired.

Pamela's Key Lime Pie

One of my all-time favorite desserts, hands down.

For the filling:

3 avocados, peeled and pitted

½ cup agave nectar

½ cup lime juice

Lime zest, to taste

Raw honey, to taste (if you want additional sweetness)

1 teaspoon coconut oil (optional)

Pinch sea salt

Blend all filling ingredients in a high-speed blender until creamy.

For the crust:

½ cup pecans, almonds or walnuts

1 cup dates, pitted

1 cup raisins

1 tablespoon pure vanilla extract

2 cups dried coconut flakes

To make the crust, start by grinding the pecans to a fine meal in a food processor. Add pitted dates, raisins and vanilla and process until the mixture reaches a dough-like consistency. Transfer dough to a bowl and work in ½ cup of the coconut flakes by hand.

Sprinkle ¾ cup of the coconut into a pie pan, then spread date/raisin/pecan mixture over the coconut. Top with the remaining coconut flakes, cover and place into the refrigerator. When crust is a bit chilled, add pie filling.

Decadent Chocomole

This is an adaptation of a recipe I got from Jason Mraz, the avocado-farming, raw-food-eating musician! My kids and father, who despise avocado, love this chocolatey treat!

1 ripe avocado, peeled and pitted
8 soft dates, pitted
2 tablespoons agave nectar
1 tablespoon vanilla extract
1 tablespoon coconut oil
1–2 tablespoons raw cacao powder or carob
A few fresh raspberries for garnish

Combine the first six ingredients in a food processor, blending until smooth and creamy. Serve in a pretty martini glass with fresh raspberries for garnish. Your friends and family will never know that you put something good for them in the pudding!

Pamela's Original Apple-Pie Salad

Another off-the-charts delicious recipe from my sweet friend Pam. This recipe was recently featured on the front page of the Living section in our local paper, the Tulsa World.

1 fresh pineapple
10 to 12 Granny Smith apples
2 cups organic raisins
2 cups shredded coconut (preferably unsweetened and unsulphured)
2 cups pecan pieces
2 tablespoons pure vanilla extract
3 tablespoons cinnamon

Split, core and peel pineapple. Place half in blender for crushed pineapple. Cut the remaining half into small chunks.

Peel, core and chop apples. If you like, soak the raisins in a small amount of water, to help them plump up, while you chop the apples. Drain raisins and combine with apples in a large bowl. Add crushed pineapple, pineapple chunks, coconut, pecan pieces and vanilla. Sprinkle cinnamon throughout.

Susan's Scrumptious Living Chocolate Cheesecake

You can delete the carob and add some fruit to this cheesecake mixture. Play with the recipe and come up with your own creations!

Prep:
Soak 3 cups cashews for an hour.

For the crust:
1½ cups almonds (I use whatever nuts I have on hand)
1 cup dates, pitted (you can use raisins instead; or half dates, half raisins)
1 heaping tablespoon carob powder

Process almonds, dates and carob powder in a food processor until the almonds are small pieces and the mixture begins to stick together. Set aside about 1 cup of the mixture to sprinkle on top of the cake before serving, and transfer the rest to a springform pan. Press evenly into pan to form crust, then put in fridge to chill.

For the filling:
3 cups soaked, drained cashews (see above)

1 cup fresh lemon juice
1 cup or less agave nectar (I used ¾ cup)
1 cup coconut oil
Splash of vanilla
2–3 tablespoons carob powder

In a food processor, blend the filling ingredients until creamy. Pour into pan over crust. Freeze cheesecake until filling firms up, then remove from freezer and let sit so you can cut it. Before serving, sprinkle with the reserved 1 cup crust topping, and garnish with fresh fruit of your choice.

Cacao Maca Ice Cream— for Raw Food Superheroes!

¼ cup raw cashew butter
2 tablespoons coconut butter
¼ cup raw cacao powder
2 tablespoons maca powder
16 medjool dates, soaked

Blend the cashew butter and coconut butter with 2–3 cups pure water to create cashew milk. Add the remaining ingredients to your blender and blend well. Pour into an ice-cream maker and process according to manufacturer's instructions, or pour into a freezable container with a lid and freeze. When your ice cream is ready, serve, salivate and enjoy!

6

Staying Detoxed in the Real World

Each of us is growing in knowledge and understanding. We're moving in a positive direction as we become empowered and act as bringers of light and change. I've recently been working with my 16-year-old daughter, Gabrielle, to teach her the importance of considering her goals and mapping her desired destinations in life. Every choice we make moves us either one step closer to or one step further away from our ultimate goals.

Now is a good time to answer these questions:

- What are your goals for your personal health and weight-loss journey?
- How do you plan to achieve those goals?
- What changes are you willing to make today to set your actions into motion and make your goals become a reality?

Even if you are successful with one or more of the four Raw Food Cleanse programs, if you don't make the necessary lifestyle shifts, you will not maintain your achievements. It's important that you make a game plan for your long-term success right now, determining what newfound strategies you want to incorporate into your daily life.

Maintaining your detox and living in vibrant health doesn't just happen. It takes a plan—and the desire to execute the plan—on your own part and even on the part of those whom your transformation will impact. As I shared in Chapter 3, you need to grab hold of the truth that you can be an example to others of what's possible. Once you seize that truth, you will *be* the influence, not the one who *is* influenced!

As I write this book, I can tell you that for many years I have been working on acquiring a taste for a lifestyle that brings lasting benefits. I haven't always gravitated naturally toward the healthiest choices, and I've had many breakdowns along the way. It is through my own personal struggles and victories that I have become the natural health advocate that I am today. It is not because I have more willpower, more resources or more motivation than you; it is because I've simply been stubborn enough to never give up. I've kept my heart open, pressing into the power of change.

The truth that has helped me the most in attaining my goals is that our thoughts and words greatly influence our relationships, self-esteem, finances, attitude, and yes, even our weight and health. Many world-renowned teachers and counselors emphasize this concept, but truly understanding and implementing it doesn't come naturally to most of us. There is a very real connection between relationships, food, focus, service and your health.

What programming in your life has been holding you back from reaching your highest potential? How are you learning to take charge of your thoughts and reprogram your thinking for a higher good? It is crucial to your optimal health that you begin to feed your body living, vibrant, easy-to-assimilate foods. It is equally important that you find a way to feed your mind positive, truthful words that bring life and joy to your soul.

You aren't reading these words by coincidence. This little book is a special delivery that was written to give you hope and point you in the right direction. Today is a new day, a fresh start and an opportunity to intentionally and lovingly take charge of what you put into your mouth and into your brain!

If you are feeling down, feeling like you are a failure or are out of control, you are not alone. Now is the time to take control of your mind and stop focusing your energy on your negative circumstances. Yes, you have the power within you to take charge of your stinkin' thinkin'! Start keeping your goals, your true heart's desire for optimal health, your list of why you are tired of failing and your list of how you are going to start succeeding constantly in front of you. Journaling is the very best thing for this. Unplug from all the lies and negativity that hold you back. Read positive things, speak and write positive words about your own life, even if you think *nobody else* believes in or respects you. The old thoughts that are no longer serving your higher good will not support you toward meeting your new, higher-resonating goals.

Another truth is that sometimes the road to real and lasting change can be lonely. When I made the commitment to change my diet and life once and for all, I had to make some other decisions that seemed to go against my nature and old desires. I had to stop spending time with people who didn't care about my ultimate well-being. You need to recognize that you may have relationships in your life today that will sabotage your efforts. These are not bad people, but they may be only looking out for ways to validate themselves and protect their own egos. The saying "misery loves company" is one you can take to the bank.

If you are an alcoholic and you make the decision to give up drinking, your common sense tells you to stay away from the bar, right? Don't drive down the street where the liquor store is if you can't handle the temptation. Likewise, don't put yourself in situations that will sabotage your success in following a diet that will help you lose weight and revitalize your life. Stop looking for empty validation from your unhealthy, stuck, overweight friends. Although they may mean well, they will gladly take you to an early grave with them.

What I'm sharing here may sound harsh, but for many of you it is going to take some radical changes in your mental, physical, spiritual and social surroundings for you to finally arrive where you want to be. And you thought this chapter was just going to tell you how to decrease your exposure to environmental and dietary toxins! It fascinates me how interconnected all of this is and how, when we set our heart and intentions on going to the next level, the needed support will manifest in ways that are both confirming and authentic. Start looking for new opportunities, road signs and the divine interventions that are just waiting to guide you, and most of all, enjoy the ride.

This chapter wouldn't be complete without some final practical tidbits of wisdom on staying physically detoxed in this world in which we live. In an effort to keep it simple and not overwhelm you, I have created a list of tips that you may want to read and re-read until they become a natural way of life for you. As I said in Chapter 2, it's impossible to avoid all environmental toxins in today's world. What you can do, however, is limit your exposure as much as possible by doing the following:

- Buy, grow and eat, as much as possible, organic produce and free-range, organic foods.
- If you eat fish, consume wild-caught fish (which is most likely not contaminated with PCBs and mercury), making sure it comes from a reputable source. Generally, large health-food distributors like Whole Foods or sustainable-friendly fishmongers have the market share of these kinds of fish.
- Avoid processed foods—they are all processed with chemicals.
- Only use natural cleaning products in your home. See the Resources section in the back of this book for recommendations.
- Switch over to natural brands of toiletries, including shampoo, toothpaste, antiperspirants and cosmetics. Again, see the Resources section for suggestions.
- As soon as you are financially able, remove any metal dental fillings. They're a major source of mercury. Be sure to have this done by a qualified biological dentist.
- Avoid using artificial air fresheners, scented dryer sheets, fabric softeners or other synthetic fragrances as they can irritate your skin and pollute the air you are breathing.
- Avoid artificial food additives of all kinds, including artificial sweeteners and MSG.
- Get plenty of safe sun exposure to boost your vitamin D levels and your immune system (you'll be better able to fight disease). I am the palest of the pale and I try to get at least 15 minutes of direct

sunlight daily without chemical sunscreens—usually before 11 a.m. or after 6 p.m.

- Find a way to test or filter your tap/well water. I now have a showerhead that filters out chlorine and my chronic problem with excessive skin itching is a thing of the past. Drinking filtered, purified, or spring water is a huge benefit to your health. Don't take my advice: research it for yourself.

- Start switching over to glass containers (like Mason jars) to store your food instead of plastic containers. The plastic might be leaching chemicals into your food.

- If you are going to eat cooked food, don't use a microwave to cook or heat it.

- Whenever possible, put your cell phone or even your cordless home phone on speaker when you're talking to someone. The less time it's up near your brain, the better!

- Minimize your exposure to sources of radiation and electromagnetic fields (EMFs). Unplug your electronics—computers, televisions and other such devices—as often as possible. Don't agree to routine x-rays unless you are in a dire health crisis. Go outside and walk barefoot to get grounded and to help neutralize and balance your compromised energy field.

7

Life Practices for Ageless Health

Any successful effort to improve one's life requires paying attention to habitual behaviors. Most of us who have struggled with weight and poor health, or are simply feeling stuck in life, have some self-sabotaging habits that are getting in the way of positive and lasting change. Lasting transformations happen in the lives of people every day, but most life makeovers include focusing your attention on crowding out defeating habits and replacing them with new, higher-resonating rituals.

As I mentioned in Chapter 4, any of the Raw Food Cleanses are best combined with the lifestyle practices shared in this chapter. Your ultimate success will be greatly enhanced when you include nurturing rituals like journaling, daily body movement, attention to your daily elimination, care for your body and skin, adequate sunlight, prayer/meditation and building a sense of service and community that will support your new and improved way of life.

Journaling

Journaling can be one of the most effective tools to help you uncover what's been working well in your life and what hasn't. It's impossible to face behaviors if we aren't aware of them, so journaling is a valuable way to explore and pay attention to what's really going on. Within the safety of your own written words, you can let your ideas and feelings flow freely, and follow them wherever they lead you. Over time your journal will give you a broader and more accurate perspective on yourself and your journey. You may be unaware of how long you have been grappling with a particular issue or challenge, but rereading entries from previous months and even years will offer you a clear perspective and allow you to see recurring themes.

Getting honest about where you are and where you want to be can become life-transforming. You get to decide who you want to be, and you can change your mind at any time. For many people, a shift in mindset begins to create tangible changes in their daily lives. But until you can allow yourself this personal freedom in real life, use journaling to try on different ways of being and expressing yourself. Write as though you are already the fearless, limitless being you aspire to be. Journaling is risk-free, private and no one but you is affected by what you write. Your journal will not resist change or pressure you to be who it thinks you ought to be!

Breathing

Breathing is so simple and fundamental, yet we often take it for granted, ignoring the power it has to affect our body, mind and spirit. Correct breathing is critically important for two reasons: it is the only means to supply our bodies and various organs with vital oxygen, and it's an important means of purging waste and toxins from the body.

Oxygen is the most vital nutrient for our bodies. It is essential to the integrity of the brain, nerves, glands and internal organs. We can do without food for weeks and without water for days, but without oxygen, we will die within a few minutes. If the brain doesn't get a proper supply of this essential nutrient, it will result in deprivation of all vital organs in the body. Oxygen is vital to our well-being, and any effort to increase the supply of oxygen, especially to the brain, will pay rich rewards.

Deep breathing is important because it makes your lymphatic system work better. The lymph system is like the body's sewage system. Every cell in your body is surrounded by lymph. Did you know that the lymphatic system is twice the size of your other circulatory system? Twice as much lymph as blood is present in our bodies, and we have twice as many lymph vessels as blood vessels. One of the keys to good health is to keep your lymphatic system open and flowing freely.

The next essential life practice for ageless health is body movement. Notice that I don't use the word *exercise*. For many of us who have struggled with weight-related issues, the utterance of the word can hold certain negative connotations. So if for no other reason than my own mental trickery, I prefer to use the term body movement.

Body Movement

Just as deep breathing brings oxygen to an often-sluggish bloodstream and clogged lymph system, simple and enjoyable body movement can and often is the catalyst that ushers in deep healing and more rapid weight loss. The options of movement are nearly limitless; however, there are particular forms of activity that will support and nurture you most effectively as you begin to focus on giving your body the attention and care it deserves.

WALKING

Walking is the most gentle, low-impact exercise that will ease you into a higher level of health and fitness while promoting an overall sense of well-being. Our bodies were created for walking, so it is clearly the most natural form of body movement. It's safe, simple and doesn't require practice, equipment or a gym membership. My doctor shared a list from the Mayo Clinic during my last checkup, outlining the health benefits associated with walking just 30 minutes per day:

- Lowering LDL cholesterol (the "bad" cholesterol)
- Raising HDL cholesterol (the "good" cholesterol)
- Lowering your blood pressure
- Reducing your risk of or managing type 2 diabetes
- Losing and managing weight
- Improving your mood
- Staying strong and fit

YOGA

Another favored form of body movement is yoga. Yoga is a cleansing practice that has proven to be extremely effective for alleviating various disorders. Yoga is also particularly helpful in these ways:

- Increasing flexibility. Yoga positions work on various joints that are often overlooked with other forms of exercise. Some people have also reported experiencing remarkable flexibility in areas of the body that have not been consciously worked upon. When done as a flow, yoga positions work in harmony to create flexibility throughout your entire body.

- Increasing lubrication in the joints, ligaments and tendons.
- Massaging of all the organs of the body. Yoga is perhaps the only form of activity that massages all the internal glands and organs of the body in such a thorough manner.
- Detoxification. By gently stretching muscles and joints as well as massaging the various organs, yoga ensures the optimum blood supply to various parts of the body. This helps flush out toxins from every nook and cranny and deliver nourishment throughout. This leads to benefits such as slower aging, increased energy and restored zest for life.
- Excellent toning of muscles that have become flaccid or weak. The repetitive stimulation and stretching sheds excess flab and creates tight, lean muscles.

REBOUNDING

Along with walking and yoga, rebounding is another form of body movement that receives my enthusiastic stamp of approval. You can practice this highly effective activity several times a day while watching television, listening to music or even talking on the phone.

When you jump on a rebounder, or mini-trampoline, the body is subjected to gravitational pulls, but unlike jogging on a hard surface, rebounding does not put any stress on your joints, knees or ankles. The jumping motion stimulates the internal organs, moves the cerebral-spinal fluid and is very beneficial for the intestines. All cells of the body become stronger in response to the motion of rebounding. The body's immune cells also become much more active, which gives them added ability to destroy viruses, bacteria and even cancer cells. Who wouldn't want to engage in a motion that directly strengthens the immune system?

Rebounding reduces body fat, which is highly beneficial in treating diabetes and many other diseases. It also provides an aerobic effect, strengthening your heart and giving your body energy when you're weary.

Along with deep breathing, walking and yoga, rebounding is an excellent way to reduce stress. I've even found myself in a trance-like state from the relaxation of the repetitive jumping, which soothes the nervous system, giving you a relaxed disposition even after you've stepped off the trampoline. The overall effect is increased resistance to environmental, physical and emotional stress. Rebounding is recommended to those who are suffering with emotional issues and depression.

Ultimately, it's up to you what form of body movement you choose. What's most important is that you find a practice that is enjoyable to you and that you can easily incorporate into your daily schedule. Many people enjoy running, swimming, hiking, biking, dancing or playing group sports like soccer, basketball or tennis. It is strictly up to you, but please understand that body movement is an integral part of living your best life now.

Elimination

Another aspect of achieving and maintaining your most vibrant health is paying attention to your elimination. I am always amazed when people tell me that they consider themselves to be regular when they only have a few bowel movements per week. As you become more in tune with your body, pay attention to what your elimination cycle is like, recognizing that you should be having *at least* one large bowel movement per day, but ultimately working toward eliminating after each meal.

If you aren't seeing approximately 18 inches of fecal matter daily, then you are likely dealing with constipation and a higher level of auto-toxicity. I know, I know . . . this subject may be taboo, but I can't in good faith write a health-related book without discussing the importance of proper elimination. I recommend educating yourself regarding ways to facilitate proper bowel cleansing to help you achieve your best health ever.

I could seriously write an entire book on this topic, but for now I will simply tell you to consider using herbal teas, enemas and colonic irrigation as part of your cleansing, healing, and weight-loss journey. If you are eating a high-raw-food diet, engaging in regular body movement, and finding ways to reduce stress, you should begin to see a dramatic improvement in your bowel pattern.

Skin Care

Many of us who have struggled with weight-related issues have also suffered from a lack of self-love. One practical way to reverse this unhealthy pattern is to nurture your body, which has been given to you as a gift. Take a bit of time each day to care for your skin. It's really quite simple and not very time-consuming to cultivate a daily skin-care ritual that will keep you looking and feeling your best well into your advanced years.

Two things I do religiously are dry-skin-brush before I shower and then apply coconut oil as a moisturizer over my entire body. First let's look at the amazing benefits of dry skin brushing.

DRY SKIN BRUSHING

- Dry skin brushing helps you shed dead skin cells, which can improve skin texture and promote cell renewal.

- Dry skin brushing increases circulation, encouraging your body's discharge of metabolic wastes, which greatly aids lymphatic drainage.

- Dry skin brushing helps to tighten the skin because it increases the flow of blood. Increasing the circulation to the skin can also lessen the appearance of cellulite.

- Dry skin brushing stimulates the lymph canals to drain toxic mucoid matter into the colon, thereby purifying the entire system. This enables the lymph to perform its house-cleaning duties: keeping the blood and other vital tissues detoxified. After several days of dry brushing, you may notice the mucous material in your stools.

- Dry skin brushing helps with muscle tone and more even distribution of fat deposits.

- Dry skin brushing rejuvenates the nervous system by stimulating nerve endings in the skin.

- Dry skin brushing helps your skin absorb nutrients by eliminating clogged pores. Healthy, breathing skin contributes to overall body health.

Individuals who sit at a computer screen all day long will particularly take pleasure in the benefits of skin brushing. People who have inactive lifestyles or desk jobs usually experience stiff necks and shoulders, and soreness that reaches even into their arms, down their spines and into their lower backs. Increased blood flow begins entering the areas brushed and you will experience an increase in electromagnetic energy that permits you to feel invigorated.

MOISTURIZE & PROTECT

Pure coconut oil is the finest natural skin moisturizer available. It leaves your skin soft and smooth with a healthy, youthful appearance. Its unique molecular structure allows it to be easily absorbed by your skin. Because it is absorbed into the cell structure of the skin, it can help protect against excessive damage from the sun. Coconut oil will keep the connective tissues in your skin strong and supple. The natural antioxidants found in coconut oil fight against free radicals that damage connective tissue and cause the skin to lose elasticity and form wrinkles.

Coconut oil also has natural antibacterial, antifungal and antimicrobial properties that provide a protective layer on your skin and can help facilitate healing of skin conditions such as rashes, acne and infections. Coconut oil contains medium-chain triglycerides, which are broken down by the good bacteria on the skin into free fatty acids. These acids in turn contribute to the acidic environment on the skin, enabling it to repel disease-causing germs.

Sunlight

The benefits of getting out into the sun have been nearly forgotten by a generation that now considers sunbathing totally taboo. There is truth that damage can be caused by staying too long in intense sunlight, increasing the risk of skin cancer, but conversely, safe sun exposure has been shown to help improve a host of chronic skin conditions including acne, eczema and psoriasis. Being in the sunshine helps build strong bones and teeth, lower cholesterol, prevent heart disease and ward off depression. And even more encouraging, many health experts believe that safe exposure to sunshine may prevent more cancers than it causes.

Sunlight triggers the body to build its own vitamin D, which is crucial not only for strong bones and healthy teeth, but for keeping the immune system fine-tuned as well. Studies have shown that exposing the body to sunlight increases the number of white blood cells or lymphocytes. These are the body's primary defense against the assault of an infection and are a significant part of your immune response to the organisms that cause illness. Vitamin D also plays a role in increasing the amount of oxygen your blood transports around the body, which boosts energy levels, sharpens your mental faculties and gives you an improved feeling of well-being.

In the early 1990s, doctors who reviewed all the medical literature examining the health risks of exposure to the sun concluded that the benefits of moderate exposure outweigh both the risk of skin cancer and premature aging. Their paper, "Beneficial Effects of Sun Exposure on Cancer Mortality," was published in *Preventive Medicine* and reported that safe sunbathing would slash the number of deaths from breast and colon cancers in America by a third.

Although it's referred to as a vitamin, D is not really a vitamin at all but a hormone-like substance that the body can only make when it gets enough sunlight. Since 90 percent of westerners now spend 90 percent of their waking time indoors, the majority of people do not get enough exposure to sunlight to make enough vitamin D. The FDA says we need 400 IU (10 mcg) of vitamin D a day to stop the body from leaching calcium from the bones.

Sunlight also triggers the increased production of the feel-good brain chemical serotonin—which, as well as controlling your sleep patterns, body temperature, and sex drive, lifts your mood and helps ward off depression.

Just 20 minutes of safe sunbathing a day is enough to get the exposure you need. The safest way to benefit from the healing powers of sunlight is to increase your exposure slowly throughout the year and to avoid burning by staying in the shade when the sun is at its most intense. To sunbathe safely, remember that frequent, short exposures are not only safer but more beneficial than an extended dose of sunlight. Also, early morning sunshine has been identified as the most beneficial.

Sleep

In the early 1900s, the average American slept 9.5 hours nightly. In 1975 that number had decreased to 7.5 hours. Now it has dropped to under 7 hours. Sixty-seven percent of Americans have sleep disorders, a 33 percent increase in the last five years. Seventy million Americans suffer from insomnia, and over 100 million Americans fail to get an adequate night's rest. When people get less than 6 to 7 hours of sleep each night, their risk for developing diseases begins to increase.

The importance of getting quality sleep every night is downplayed in our super busy, late-night culture. Going to sleep before midnight is almost unheard of by a large majority of the population, yet our immune system functions optimally if we go to sleep by 10 p.m. As we sleep, physical repair takes place between approximately 10 p.m. and 2 a.m. Our immune cells patrol our bodies, eliminating cancer cells, bacteria, viruses, and other harmful agents. Then from about 2 a.m. to 6 a.m., we enter a stage of psychic regeneration. During this time, the brain releases chemicals that enhance our immune system. Throughout the night, we experience rapid eye movement (REM) sleep states and non-REM sleep, alternating between light sleep and deep dream states. This is how we process the mental and emotional events of the previous day and restore our minds for the day ahead.

Most people need a minimum of seven or eight hours of sleep to accomplish these tasks. Without adequate sleep, the immune system is hard-pressed to keep up with its damage control. This creates the opportunity for disease to take hold. Additionally, if cortisol is elevated at night, which can happen if you are anxious, these immune functions can become compromised, which eventually leads to weight gain, illness and disease. Here is a list of reasons sufficient sleep is so critical for sustained weight loss and vital for you if you're to find your own optimum health:

SLEEP KEEPS YOUR HEART HEALTHY   Heart attacks and strokes are more common during the early morning hours. This fact may be explained by the way sleep affects the blood vessels. Lack of sleep is associated with the increase of blood pressure and cholesterol, both risk factors for heart disease and stroke. Your heart will be healthier if you get between 7 and 9 hours of sleep each night.

SLEEP MAY HELP PREVENT CANCER   Those who work the late shift have a higher risk for breast and colon cancer. Researchers believe this is caused by differing levels of melatonin in people who are exposed to light at night. Light exposure reduces the level of melatonin, a hormone that both makes us sleepy and is thought to protect against cancer. Melatonin appears to suppress the growth of tumors. Be sure that your bedroom is dark to help your body produce the melatonin it needs.

SLEEP REDUCES STRESS   If your body is sleep deficient, it goes into a state of stress. The body's functions are put on high alert, which causes an increase in blood pressure and the production of stress hormones. Higher blood pressure increases your risk for heart attacks and strokes. The stress hormones also, unfortunately, make it harder for you to sleep.

SLEEP REDUCES INFLAMMATION   An increase in stress hormones raises the level of inflammation in your body, which creates more risk for heart conditions, cancer and diabetes. Inflammation is thought to be one of the causes of the deterioration of your body as you age.

SLEEP MAKES YOU MORE ALERT   Of course, a good night's sleep makes you feel energized and alert the next day. Being plugged in and active not only feels great, it also increases your chances for another good night's sleep. When you wake up feeling refreshed, you feel like going out into the day, being active and engaged in your world. You'll sleep better the next night and increase your daily energy level.

SLEEP BOLSTERS YOUR MEMORY   It's not fully known why we sleep and dream, but a process called memory consolidation occurs during sleep. While your body may be resting, your brain is busy processing your day, making connections between experiences, sensory input, feelings and memories. Your dreams and deep sleep are an important time for your brain to make memories and links. Getting more quality sleep will help you remember and process things better.

SLEEP MAY HELP YOU LOSE WEIGHT   Researchers have also found that people who sleep less than seven hours per night are more likely to be overweight or obese. It is thought that the lack of sleep impacts the balance of hormones in the body that affect appetite. The hormones ghrelin and leptin, important for the regulation of appetite, have been found to be disrupted by lack of sleep.

SLEEP MAY REDUCE YOUR RISK FOR DEPRESSION
Sleep impacts many of the chemicals in your body, including serotonin. People with a deficiency in serotonin are more likely to suffer from depression. You can help to prevent depression by making sure you are getting the right amount of sleep, between 7 and 9 hours each night.

SLEEP HELPS THE BODY MAKE REPAIRS Sleep is a time for your body to repair damage caused by stress, ultraviolet rays and other harmful exposures. Your cells produce more protein while you are sleeping. These protein molecules form the building blocks for cells, allowing them to repair damage.

Feeding the Spirit

For me, one of the most powerful aspects of my total health journey has been "to be still and know the voice of God" and to learn about my purpose in this life and how to flourish in that purpose. Choosing to live a life that includes prayer and meditation helps connect you to a listening God. As you begin to listen to that still, small voice within, you naturally start gravitating toward fulfilling your purpose on this planet, becoming transformed more each day into the person you were created to be.

"Spirituality is an essential dimension of being human. and as much a part of us as our bodies and minds," shares Jonathan Ellerby, PhD, author of *Return to the Sacred*. "It's not a matter of whether or not you're spiritual, but of what kind of spiritual personality you have." I recommend Ellerby's book as a helpful starting place if you feel detached from your spirituality.

I have seen that in the place of the Spirit, all things become possible; healing and weight loss can occur no matter how severe or long-standing the situation. This is the place of miracles, where the body does what it was designed to do—heal. Just as a cut naturally heals in time, without thought, without action, without any effort, so can disease heal when all the blockages, imbalances, and toxins have been released from body, mind, and emotions.

THE SIGNIFICANCE OF PRAYER/MEDITATION/STILLNESS

Prayer is the simple act of communicating or communing with God. Most of your time in communion can be spent listening to the voice spoken into your heart. Holy scriptures teach that you can begin to clearly know God's voice rather than the voice of your mind, your emotions, or the world system when you begin to seek Him with all of your heart. For me, this happened when I recognized the end of my own ideas, strength and ability to change. As I became humbled and still, in a place of fasting and prayer, the direction and empowerment for change started to happen.

Even if you don't consider yourself to be a spiritual or religious person, there is much research that shows prayer and meditation to be hugely beneficial in overcoming life's most stubborn challenges, like disease and obesity. Here are some statistics:

- Many physicians recommend meditation to prevent and control pain in patients suffering from chronic illnesses or conditions such as heart disease, AIDS, cancer and infertility.
- Prayer can restore balance to those afflicted with mental conditions such as depression, hyperactivity and attention deficit disorder (ADD).
- For 30 years, medical research has shown that prayer can reduce emotional stress.

- Prayer can "reset" the brain to change behavior (for example, reducing one's tendency toward road rage).
- Those who pray are generally healthier and live longer. They have lower blood pressure and lower incidence of stroke and heart disease. They are less likely to smoke or drink and tend to get sick less often.
- The authors of the *Handbook of Religion and Health* document nearly 1,200 studies done on the effects of prayer on health. Here are some of those statistics:
  - Hospitalized people who never attended church have an average stay that is three times longer than people who attended regularly.
  - Heart patients were 14 times more likely to die following surgery if they did not participate in a religion.
  - Elderly people who never or rarely attended church had a stroke rate double that of people who attended regularly.
  - In Israel, religious people had a 40 percent lower death rate from cardiovascular disease and cancer.

The author of *The Blue Zones*, Dan Buettner, writes: "The simple act of regularly attending a religious service or ceremony seems to be a common thread among cultures with the longest life spans. It doesn't matter what your faith practice is—attending a religious service—even once a month, seems to have positive effects on overall health and happiness. A study in the Journal of Health and Social Behavior followed over 2,500 people for seven and a half years and discovered that *those who attended regular religious services (one to three times per month) had a longer life expectancy than those who did not.*"

All of this comes as no surprise to those who have an active faith, but for those who do not, perhaps these facts will open you up to considering your own spirituality, not as just a concept, something on paper, or a religious myth, but as real. When God becomes real for you, life is never the same again and prayer is not a waste of time, but a fountain of new life.

To begin, the practice of meditative prayer should last for at least 15 minutes each day, as it's hard to quiet the mind and body in less than that amount of time. Praying with a spiritual book or with scriptures can be very helpful. Finding a quiet place where you can be alone and undistracted by noise or cell phones is key. Begin by asking God, as you know him, to help you focus during this time of prayer. God has no problem being with us, although we often have the problem of being distant from God. Be quiet for a few moments to listen and think about God. Think about whom you are addressing. Dwell on this thought for a while. If you have a good imagination, visualize being in His presence: imagine the two of you talking and walking together. Imagine him touching you gently, smiling and saying, "Peace be with you." What is happening inside you? How are you feeling? Allow forgiveness and love to flow over and through you at this time.

Because so many of us have been wounded by religion, its people and its dogmas, this exercise is a meaningful way to reconnect with our own spirituality in a personal and intimate way. There is much healing and freedom in this practice. During these precious times of spiritual awakening, you can start to believe that it is God's perfect will for you to be made whole; all you have to do is receive.

Community

A support group can be a great resource for people with health issues and for those who are hoping to lose weight permanently. This is likely the reason that Weight Watchers has been the world's most successful approach to lasting weight loss. The emotional support and encouragement of like-minded people can be so significant when trying to achieve your best health ever. Look for opportunities to join raw food groups in your area or online groups that will allow you to share your achievements, recipes, ideas and even your challenges. The camaraderie of others who have the same goal can help you avoid pitfalls such as emotional eating and bingeing. (In the Resource section at the back of this book, you'll find information on a suggested web-based community of support for raw foodists.)

Finding new healthy relationships, either online or in person, will help you with challenges such as remaining accountable, staying within your dietary budget, overcoming cravings and getting past plateaus. Whenever you want to share tips, get support or simply chat about weight- and health-related challenges and successes, this type of community can provide an outlet for you.

When I decided to write this book, I created an online research group to help collect data for my writing. I had no way of knowing that this online community would evolve into something so beneficial for both the research project and for all of those who participated. This online community was blessed with individuals who were on the same wavelength and committed to similar goals. Although the group started out retaining some anonymity, it quickly evolved into a safe haven where we were all able to support one another openly, with fewer inhibitions.

I think you'll find the community research that we accumulated over an 11-week period one of the most intriguing, life-changing parts of this book. Get comfortable, grab a box of tissues and get ready to open your heart to the stories of real-life superheroes in the pages to come.

8

Real Stories from Raw Food Superheroes

This chapter is composed of stories from the final 65 participants of the Raw Food Cleanse Experiment. I conducted the 11-week program to gather evidence supporting the claims of this book. In the pages that follow, you'll find inspirational, motivational, encouraging stories, all from real people who've overcome many health and weight issues by changing their diets and their lives.

• • •

Shortly after I signed the contract with Ulysses Press to write *Raw Food Cleanse*, I hosted a dinner party at my home. Jen Hoppa attended as a guest of one of my closest friends. I had met Jen a couple of times before at local raw food events. When I shared with the dinner guests that I had been commissioned to write a book outlining four specific raw food cleanses for individuals wanting to restore their health and lose weight, Jen quickly offered to be a guinea pig for my cleanse research. In addition to being a longtime vegetarian and vibrant new-experience seeker, Jen had a bit of weight she wanted to lose, so she was instantly motivated to try the program.

That night over dinner-party conversation, I realized others around the globe might also like to be part of the experiment. A few days later I put a video on YouTube and RawFu, a raw food social-networking site, asking for volunteers to participate in the research for this book. Within 24 hours, I had nearly 200 e-mails from people who hoped to be chosen for such a project. Needless to say, I was thrilled, but I was also overwhelmed. Because of the time sensitivity, I had to pick my guinea pigs immediately, as the research would need to begin in a matter of days. I had to turn away hundreds of interested project volunteers, all people just like you, eager to try anything to lose weight and find their optimal health.

Over the course of the following 11 weeks, many participants became inactive or were removed from the research for a variety of reasons, but in the end, 65 participants successfully completed the program. These participants lost a combined total of over 900 pounds, and the individual results, which I am about to share with you, are staggering. But even more interesting, the friendships and connections that developed within the research group reveal how vital a sense of community and camaraderie can be in helping you reach your personal goals.

Back to Jen: Not only did she successfully complete the 11-week Raw Food Cleanse Experiment, she also talked her very hesitant, skeptical parents into joining her. The Hoppa family's story is one that will stir, motivate and inspire you.

The Hoppas—Bill, 52; Katy, 51; and Jen, 24

Tulsa, Oklahoma

Jen made the decision to become a vegetarian at age 12, much to the dismay of her parents. They questioned her reasons for such an unexpected pronouncement and tried to convince her how difficult and complicated such a life might be at school and in social situations. Their concerns continued to grow as Jen became more determined about her decision. Where would she get her protein and adequate nutrition, especially when she was so young and still growing developmentally?

After much debate and many long family discussions, Jen made her final choice, and she has maintained a vegetarian lifestyle ever since. Her parents have continued to lovingly support their daughter's lifestyle choice, but they did not adopt a vegetarian diet themselves. Recently, when Jen approached them about her new raw food diet, the eyebrows raised once again. Katy shares her experience:

> Our daughter Jen first started incorporating raw food into her diet after joining a local group, Real Food Tulsa, which facilitates raw food potlucks and holds monthly meetings on the lifestyle. Even though she was only getting her feet wet with this way of eating, I began seeing amazing results in her within a short period of time. I have never been a vegetable eater, and the thought of eating raw vegetables was less than appealing to me. Months later, Jen told me that she was embarking on another, more intense raw-food diet, but this time as an experiment for a friend who was writing a book on the subject. For some reason, I listened with more interest.

I was quickly approaching menopause and had gained 40 pounds over the last three years. Nothing I did seemed to get the weight off. As the Raw Food Cleanse Experiment kickoff date grew closer, I wondered if *I* could possibly eat a raw food diet. As a last-minute whim—and I do mean last-minute—my husband and I decided to support Jen and committed to *try* to eat raw foods for three days. I thought that if Bill and I could just lose a few pounds and feel a bit better it might be worth the hell we were sure to experience.

After only three days of 100 percent raw eating, I was hooked. Daily I made one of Penni's cleansing smoothies with chia seeds, coconut oil and lots of greens and fruit. Green Smoothies usually made up two meals of our day, but we ate snacks of highly nutritious foods and a raw evening meal. For the first time in my life I was never hungry. Sugar, carb and chocolate cravings were gone. Since we began eating this way, our lives have been revolutionized by a raw food diet. We are eating the best food of our lives and living our best life ever.

Katy Hoppa lost 25 pounds in 10 weeks. In her final evaluation, she shares that her overall health has greatly improved, her energy level has greatly increased, she feels more balanced in her emotions and has had a clearing of long-term "brain fog." Other improvements include smoother, clearer, glowing skin, stronger nails and decreased hair loss. She was also motivated to add walking to her daily health regime. Finally, Katy adds:

I now see my high-raw-foods diet as a lifestyle that I will carry throughout my entire life. A very close friend who is a medical doctor asked me one question after learning that I had begun a 100 percent raw food diet:

"Can you eat this way forever?" He said he always asks this question of his patients when they talk about diets and losing weight. He asked this during my first week of eating raw and my answer was "Let's wait and see." Now, after 11 weeks, my answer is unequivocally, "YES!"

Katy's husband, Bill, also had a dramatic experience with the Raw Food Cleanse. At 52 years old, 5'7" and 235 pounds, Bill was hesitant about this way of eating, yet he too was ready for a change. At the beginning of the experiment, he viewed eating a raw food diet as extreme and "counter-cultural," certainly not something one could realistically maintain for any length of time.

Read along as Bill shares his experiences:

The past 10 weeks have been such a positive experience because of the absence of cravings. Both weight loss and the overall health benefits such as lowered blood pressure, tighter, firmer skin, more energy, strength, endurance and improved concentration were noticeable in a short amount of time. It just seemed that these improvements were automatic benefits that simply happened by themselves as a result of the lifestyle change. Every other diet I had tried in the past gave me a sense of being on a temporary, deprivation-oriented, unnatural, forced way of eating.

This has been one of the top five most transformational experiences of my life! For the first time since emerging from my mother's womb, I am not preoccupied and controlled by food: hunger, cravings, addictions, and all the other horrible consequences of the standard American diet. I thought people who ate this way were unnecessarily fanatical and misinformed. Through personal education and experience, my eyes have been opened and my life has been transformed. I can now see, taste and feel the positive difference in real, whole, natural, organic and raw foods. In the past, every moment was focused on when I would enjoy my next morsel. Now I use every morsel to enhance my ability to enjoy my next moment. Tectonic plates have shifted: I now eat to live rather than live to eat.

Since Katy, Jen and I did this experiment as a team, it has brought us closer together as a family. The outcome of this bonding experience is equally as significant as the 32 pounds I lost in the process. Now my primary concern is relationship rather than food. One of my new life missions is to bring raw food to real people.

Of course by now you must be wondering what happened with Jen. Even though Jen had been a vegetarian for over half her life, that didn't mean she kept a meticulously healthy watch over everything she ate. As many know, it's possible to be a vegetarian and still not be totally healthy. Here are some of her observations from the experiment:

Prior to trying the Raw Food Cleanse, I was taking a lot of naps and feeling generally sluggish. I would get tired at work, which would affect my performance and dampen my mood. Since I started eating a very high raw foods diet, I now have improved clarity and focus. Although I was not taking it regularly, I did have a prescription for Adderall to help with my ADD tendencies. This way of eating helped me to focus with more intent and motivation. I think I've taken one nap in the past three months. I also sleep better and feel more rejuvenated after sleeping than I did before.

Another benefit was an improvement in bowel function. I've generally never had a lot of BMs, having one or none at all per day. This has always bothered me and although I've tried "increasing my fiber" many a time, I've never had changed results. Eating a high raw diet increased my BMs to a comfortable level of regularity that I hadn't experienced before. It has helped me to feel much lighter and more "clean."

I think the 80/20 model is ideal for my body and perfect for dealing with cravings, social events and traveling. If you try to do 100 percent raw all the time, then any slip-up is interpreted as a failure. But with the 80/20 diet, if you end up only eating 80 percent raw one day, there is no guilt. If you eat more than 80 percent raw, there is a feeling of accomplishment. The 80/20 model is really helpful for long-term success. If something is not attainable, people will not do it. I feel so amazing after eating a high-raw diet, there is no way I'm going to let myself relapse back into a world of fatigue and poor health. I want raw to be a lifestyle for me. I see it as the perfect way to maintain my weight loss.

Jen lost 14 pounds during the 11 weeks that she participated in the research experiment. The Hoppas continue to maintain this healthy way of eating along with following many of the Life Practices for Ageless Health (see Chapter 7). Jen is maintaining her weight loss and Bill and Katy continue to lose weight toward their goals.

Dawn Maiorana, 42
Pleasant Valley, New York

Since making the decision to eat a high raw diet, including Green Smoothies and juicing, I feel like I've taken my body and my life back. The fog has lifted from my brain and I feel vibrant, happy and excited to live each day! I have had annoying spotting in between periods for years and years. Since I've been committed to the Raw Food Cleanse, I've hardly experienced any symptoms at all. Also, I used to have very heavy, clotty periods with severe cramps, but during my last cycle I noticed things were much less painful and not nearly as heavy. This breakthrough and the 14 pounds I lost are reason enough to continue to eat a high-raw-foods diet for the rest of my life—it just feels like the natural thing to do.

Anna H., 35
Barrie, Ontario

I've always struggled with my health. As a child, I generally spent one to two weeks in the hospital every year with pneumonia, tonsillitis or a horrible bout of the flu. I've also been challenged with a few autoimmune disorders. I added to the complexity of my compromised constitution by taking up a few destructive habits in my early adult years, like smoking, caffeine consumption, undereating, overeating or just eating poorly, not getting enough sleep, and burning the candle at both ends. Over time, the cumulative effects of my challenged health and lifestyle choices caught up with me and it became clear that I had to make some serious changes.

Food seemed to be the most obvious aspect to change, so I started there. However, it wasn't easy and it didn't just happen overnight. When you start caring about what you eat, it's an act of self-love and self-preservation, which ultimately spills over into other areas of your life. Changing my diet has not only helped me to lose 12 pounds so far, it has also brought such relief. I now feel as if I have found real answers and a way out of the vicious cycle I was in. Not only has my physical health improved, but my mental well-being has been greatly enhanced as well.

My choices have affected everyone around me. My children now love smoothies and love to taste different raw food recipes. They have even started to pay attention to how different foods make them feel. My husband has started asking me questions about his health and has finally agreed to go in for his *first ever* physical. I hosted a dinner party for all of my friends that included a number of raw food dishes, and they were amazed at how delicious everything was. I hope to continue to be an ambassador of positive change within my sphere of influence, sharing the message of how foods affect your health and healing.

Barbara, 45

Silver Spring, Maryland

The Raw Food Cleanse has brought so many positive changes into my life. Saying goodbye to dairy products and gluten-containing foods has been a huge aspect of my restored health. No more gas or bloating, yea! Also, my blood pressure went from being borderline to being well within the normal range. Incorporating more raw foods into my diet has helped me to love myself more, putting me in closer touch with the world around me. They say you are what you eat, and I believe that is so true. Before I learned about raw foods, I was rushed, always choosing packaged foods that were full of artificial ingredients. Now I appreciate nature's bounty and find joy in something as simple as a fresh tomato! Every time I choose to eat raw, I'm deciding to be kind to my body. This is a huge breakthrough. It's like my diet before was self-abusive. I'm truly grateful to have found this life-restoring path.

Misti Young, 38
Salem, Oregon

Being part of the Raw Food Cleanse Experiment has been such a positive experience for me. I'm still shaking my head in wonder that I even joined a group like this at all, let alone actually participated! I have always been a lurker type, but in this group and with this experiment, I have really put myself out there in ways I never thought were possible for me. Eating a raw food diet, being part of all the honesty and watching the personal videos from others has given me a new confidence in myself. I now perceive myself as someone others would want to talk to, know or look at, and it's not just about the 10 pounds I lost. It amazes me that this kind of transformation can happen in a person's life both inside and out just by eating living foods! My results were so quick, too. I now tell everyone I can about what eating fresh, organic raw foods can do for them. Green smoothies are the BOMB!

Afsheen Mayhai, 23, and
Hannah Mayhai, 25 (husband and wife)
Burlington, Iowa
Hannah said:

It is through raw food that I've finally started to get my life back. I had a baby 18 months ago and the postpartum depression and weight gain really affected me. I had never been over 200 pounds before, and by the time I found the Raw Food Cleanse opportunity I was pushing 250 pounds. The weight gain and depression caused my friendships to start diminishing because I had gone into a shell. Not only was my social life affected, but so was my schooling.

Now that I have lost 15 pounds, I'm encouraged and actually feel like getting back into life. My mind was so foggy before, but now it's much clearer and I'm doing so much better. Eating this way has given me hope and I am starting to see the light!

From Afsheen:

This experience has been really positive. All of the discussions on a variety of topics were really helpful. I now have a better idea of what this is all about and what it means to eat and live a raw, holistic lifestyle. I feel like a kid who has just learned to feed himself for the first time.

Andrea Crossman, 38
Brooklyn, New York

This group was heaven sent. As a holistic nurse and cofounder of a love-infused social entrepreneurship venture called Lovemore, I was deeply bothered when I began to realize that I was not in alignment with my own mantra, "love more," in some fundamental ways. I had stopped the exercise I loved, put back on 40 pounds that I was oh-so-proud to have lost a few years ago, and my social life had all but ground to a halt as I struggled with not feeling right in my skin or in my spirit. It was in that place that I stumbled upon Penni's open call for guinea pigs. Serendipity like this is not to be ignored. This raw connection back to my soul was masterminded by the cosmos, of that I have no doubt.

The love and support I found in the group was amazing and the accountability has been huge for me. Another critical factor in my success was that I viewed this experiment as focused not on weight loss, but actually on love and health, with weight loss as the natural outcome. That mindset totally worked for me.

It's so wonderful to be enjoying my food, feeling the vibrations of being well-fed and completely nourished, while still being able to eat foods I consider to be treats, and while losing weight at the same time. This weight-loss experiment has been a revelation for me. I don't feel deprived—with the sense of orneriness, depression or wanting to act out that comes along with deprivation. In fact, I actually feel very well-loved as a result of getting to have all of these beautiful, fresh, delicious foods in abundance every day.

Andrea lost nearly 30 pounds during our Raw Food Cleanse Experiment and her delightful presence made us all feel *loved more*.

Debbie Dise, 54
Tahlequah, Oklahoma

Thirty years ago I was introduced to raw foods by Ann Wigmore. The information in her books just made sense to me and changed my life for the better. I grew indoor greens and made Rejuvelac and could f eel how important live enzyme-enriched foods were for my body.

I went on to become a licensed midwife and saw how important good nutrition was for pregnant moms and their growing babies. Some of the healthiest moms and babies I helped birth were high-raw vegan families. I went on to get my license as a body worker and colon hydrotherapist and started learning a lot about degenerative diseases and how the standard American diet was contributing to mass amounts of pain and suffering. What people were eating was literally killing them.

By the time I learned about the Raw Food Cleanse Experiment, I was totally vested and ready to be a part. What a blessing of divine timing and guidance it has been for the past 11 weeks. Many have mentioned that I am looking younger and I've noticed that my skin is less wrinkled. Eleven pounds less makes me look thinner, healthier and more youthful.

So here I am right now in this present moment, emerging into higher levels of vibrant health and well-being, knowing that I have a sisterhood and brotherhood of raw food friends supporting me all the way. Plant-based eating is my future, and it's essential for a peaceful, healthy planet.

Cindy Cummins, 48
Minneapolis, Minnesota, and Portland, Oregon

I've done many cleanses over the years, but I prefer the Raw Food Cleanse, which allows me to lose weight, maintain the weight loss and keep my energy levels high. In the past I've had to starve myself, whereas with this approach I could eat delicious, satisfying meals. I was able to detoxify my system yet stay focused while working and exercising regularly. Joint pain and gallbladder pain of eight-plus years was gone. I was also amazed to get my metabolism back up and running without the use of unhealthy exercise stimulants!

Losing twelve pounds is awesome, but as my journal entries show, I released stuck emotions on many levels. For example, I was unaware that I was chronically blaming other people. This topic came up one day on the website; combined with the dietary detox, something clicked. I feel as though I moved a chunk of resentment out of my being! This is a long-term lifestyle choice. I'm a raw food lover for life!

Stacey Bradford, 29
Seattle, Washington

I feel so vibrant eating raw! It's been so interesting because I considered myself to be fairly healthy before I started this cleanse. However, as I began eating more and more raw foods, some of the things I considered to be normal about myself started to disappear. For example, I thought it was normal to have itchy skin. When I realized that I had been creating the itchiness with my diet, I was stunned. My skin cleared up, my acid reflux went away, the pain in my knees reduced and my hair and nails grew longer and more luxurious. How powerful is that?

During the experiment I chose to do water and juice feasting, which helped me get over my fear of not snacking. I had always thought that I had low blood sugar because I had to eat every two or three hours so I wouldn't get lightheaded or run down. I believed this about myself because I grew up hearing my mom always saying that about herself. I didn't realize it before, but I had actually conditioned myself to think that this was just normal and "this is just how I am." Now I can go for many hours between meals and be just fine. Doing the water/juice fasts has been such a powerful revelation for me because now I know I'll be fine to just wait until I can have some fruit or veggies. I don't have to feed my body junk out of unfounded panic.

Even though my husband's not raw, or vegan or even a vegetarian, he is still totally supportive of me. I will definitely continue to eat a high raw diet. Even though I lost 14 pounds, it's not about the weight loss for me, this is now my lifestyle and I don't see that ever changing. This is not a fad diet; it's just who I am.

Francine Rodriguez, 52
Tampa, Florida

I've known about the benefits of the raw food diet for years now. During the Raw Food Cleanse my complexion improved, growing brighter and clearer. I experienced higher energy levels and my thinking was much sharper. Eating raw is a lifestyle choice for me now; it's what Spirit is pushing me to do.

Mauri Whalen, 44
Portland, Oregon

Before doing the Raw Food Cleanse, I was having mini hot flashes. WHAT? I'm only 44! I'd wake up in the middle of the night all sweaty, or during the day, just out of nowhere I'd get really hot. Not pleasant at all! About three weeks into this experiment I stopped having hot flashes altogether. Call it a coincidence that they are gone or call it raw food helping my perimenopausal symptoms—I am convinced it's raw!

Throughout the experiment I drank about two quarts of Green Juice each day and ate a 90 percent raw diet. I lost almost 14 pounds, and it feels great to be in control of my health. I laugh because I am now addicted to Green Juice just like I used to be addicted to Diet Coke! This is a way of life for me now. It has been nothing but positive and I plan to live this way for the rest of my life.

Deepak Rajanikanth, 26
Bangalore, India

Before the Raw Food Cleanse, my diet was about 5 percent raw. When I decided to join the experiment, I expected to last about two weeks. But I ended up surviving the full 11 weeks and now my life is on a healthy course. I now know that I can live on a complete diet of raw foods without depending on cooked or processed items.

My friends and family totally supported me on this as well. They even began to add raw foods in their diets. The results began to show quickly for me: detoxing created glowing, healthy skin and the feeling of being much lighter. There were days when I felt as though I would lose hope and give in, but my fellow members within the community continued to cheer me on and that kept me going. I loved the new recipes, smoothies and even the chia seeds made my raw-food intake tastier and more fun.

I lost 18 unwanted pounds in 11 weeks. Accomplishing this has helped me to pursue other hobbies I enjoy, like dancing and cycling. My confidence level in the way I speak and walk has really improved. I believe that this way of eating will always be a part of my lifestyle from now on.

Deborah Blank, 55
Carmichael, California

I am just your average 55-year-old female trying to get by with as few aches and pains and health issues as possible. The Raw Food Cleanse Experiment reaffirmed to me that Green Smoothies are the perfect food. They are totally healthy, nutritious and satisfying. I've also just gotten into juicing. I like that it's an instant jolt of pure plant goodness.

In the last 11 weeks my rosacea cleared significantly (I stopped all prescription meds for it), I've had less body odor, I've had no new MS flares and the residual symptoms are slightly less, my normal morning ankle and foot pain has disappeared, and my seasonal allergies aren't present, even during a terrible allergy season. I'm sleeping through the night, I'm less fatigued and I have high energy when I'm at the gym, walking or hiking. My blood pressure is down, my hair is shedding less, and I'm no longer having issues with constipation and indigestion. I was also having horrendous periods, but now I have very light ones and big gaps in between. I'm starting menopause so this is expected, but prior to this experiment I was having serious anemic-making periods.

I lost 13 pounds and 22 inches and know that raw (80 percent) is the way to go for me. I have dabbled on and off for a couple of years and cannot tell you how much better I feel on raw than off. If I can just keep all of this in mind, I will never be tempted to stray far from raw.

Kerry, 40
Salem, Oregon

I've struggled with fibromyalgia for over 15 years, and since I started eating raw last January, my muscle soreness is much improved. I'm convinced that my body is putting all this newfound energy into helping me feel better. Speaking of energy, I've earned the reputation now as the Energizer bunny because I just keep going and going. It must be all the raw foods that have me so powered up! Since I've been on the Raw Food Cleanse I've dropped eight pounds and my ulcerative colitis has gone bye-bye!

Teri Wayne, 56
Knoxville, Tennessee

Since starting the Raw Food Cleanse I have been more observant about what I have been putting into my mouth. My diet consisted of only about 25 percent raw foods when I began this experiment. I thought that what I was eating was healthy, but now I realize it wasn't all that great.

Because I have hypothyroidism, it has been a battle to lose weight, no matter what or how hard I tried. On most diets I would actually gain weight. With the Raw Food Cleanse, the nearly 20-pound weight loss was painless. I have not been starving myself and the weight is just falling off. This experience has been such a blessing. I will certainly continue to follow this dietary lifestyle because it's easy and I really feel great.

Aimee K., 39

Lewisburg, Pennsylvania

I completely understand why people might be put off at first by the idea of eating raw. For most of us who grew up on TV dinners, white bread and fast food, eating raw seems like a completely foreign concept, when in fact it is the oldest and most natural way to eat.

My introduction to raw foods came years ago while living in California. Only 25 years old at the time, I was still living the party life when I took a job as a server at a raw food restaurant called Garden Taste. Unfortunately I missed the call and didn't feel a need to make any changes to my then standard American diet, but thankfully, a seed had been planted.

Ten years later when I was living in Oregon, my concern for the environment led me to join a group called the Northwest Earth Institute, a grassroots organization with programs emphasizing individual responsibility in adopting a more sustainable lifestyle. There I learned the benefits of eating organic, seasonal and locally grown foods. This new knowledge, coupled with the fact that I was becoming a first-time mom, led me to begin making healthier food choices, though my diet still consisted of mostly cooked foods, including meats.

After my son's birth, I fell into the common trap of thinking being a "good mother" meant sacrificing my own needs. So, while I focused a lot of my energy on making sure my son got the best nutrition possible, I failed to make my own health a priority. In two years, I gained over 50 pounds and acquired a long list of aches, pains and inflammatory problems.

When my health issues began noticeably interfering with my life, I knew I needed to change. Innately I felt that the best path to optimal health and wellness for me was to add more living foods to my diet. While I dabbled in eating raw a few times in recent months, I lacked direction and needed help transitioning. Then, as fate would have it, I was given the opportunity to be a guinea pig in the Raw Food Cleanse.

Penni's guidance has made a huge difference in my life. Just the simple act of beginning my day with 32 ounces of pure, alkaline, mineral-rich water helped me shift away from my habit of getting up in the morning and immediately doing for others. It's a gift I now give myself each morning.

Although I was not one of the biggest weight-loss stories within the group, I noticed tremendous positive changes within weeks of converting to a high-raw diet. Most of my ailments are now gone or drastically improved, my skin is glowing, my overall mood is brighter and my confidence greater. There is no doubt that I will continue to eat this way, for myself and for the planet.

Jodi Clark, 44
La Quinta, California

Although there is certainly a learning curve when it comes to transitioning from a typical American diet to one that is high in raw foods, I found the education and community support invaluable as I participated in the Raw Food Cleanse Experiment. Within just a couple of weeks, eating this new way became easier and I could actually feel the difference. I no longer crave junk food or sweets and my taste for animal protein has diminished almost entirely. I look forward to my meals and see them as a true source of life and energy for my body.

I'm thrilled to have lost 14 pounds during the experiment, but am even more encouraged that my gallbladder symptoms are completely gone. My chronic fatigue and fibromyalgia pains decreased and my mental clarity improved dramatically. All previous symptoms of PMS, cramps, bloating, breast tenderness, extreme fatigue and nausea are gone. I view this as only the beginning of my newfound life. Eating this way will certainly be a lifestyle choice from now on.

Wendy Agee, 34
Mentor, Ohio

Even though Wendy had already embraced a raw foods lifestyle before joining our research group, she made a more intense commitment during the 11-week experiment. She upped her daily intake from about 75 percent to 90 percent raw and she added regular walking and biking to her routine. Wendy was able to get below 200 pounds for the first time in years, losing 15 pounds and 12 inches. Being a raw foodist is just who Wendy is at this point; there is no turning back now!

Aimee Bittinger, 30

Seattle, Washington

Since I started the Raw Food Cleanse, people say I look better and less tired, and I agree. Even though I was eating raw before the cleanse, I tried some new approaches like juice fasting. I was really intimidated by the idea, but upon hearing other people's stories and having Penni's support, I embarked on the five days recommended. It was not easy for me. I've given up many foods in my life, and it's never been easy, but giving up all food for even a short while was really a hard concept for me. Within a short time I began to realize my emotional attachment to food. Since I've had food allergies and restrictions for over 10 years, I've always been worried if I didn't eat enough I might starve. Through juicing, I realized I can survive with less and learn to appreciate what I have! After my juice feast, people commented on my skin being smoother and softer and my eyes being clearer.

The number-one best change that I implemented during the 11 weeks was drinking 32 ounces of water first thing every morning. It helped me so much, and I plan to keep this as a habit for life. On this cleanse, I gained lots of information and skills that I will continue to use. I will continue to eat a mostly raw diet. It seems like the perfect way to maintain weight and to be healthier overall.

Anita Repp, 63

Tulsa, Oklahoma

I doubled my raw food percentage during the Raw Food Cleanse Experiment. I noticed that eating this way brought an enormous amount of mental clarity after I got my system cleansed from sugar and processed foods. I plan to continue to eat a higher, healthier level of raw foods, eliminating those foods that I know don't encourage health or add longevity to my life.

T. Larson, 47
Moorhead, Minnesota

Before I started eating a raw foods diet I had a multitude of ailments. Nothing specifically life-threatening, but I had irritable bowel syndrome, acne, dry skin, allergies, migraines, PMS, borderline obsessive-compulsive disorder, an ulcer since I was 13, arthritis, carpal tunnel syndrome . . . and probably more things that I am forgetting now because they are gone. Since changing my diet, I have not had to take medication for anything. As long as I stay raw, the PMS and allergies are kept at bay. My bottle of ulcer medication has collected much dust. I sleep more soundly and wake more rested even on less sleep. Acne and dry skin patches only start to reappear if I return to my old patterns of eating.

Being 47 years old, I was starting to see gross granny skin on my feet, elbows and knees—you know the chicken skin I'm referring to. All of that is gone, and without having to slather on lotions or creams. I've also lost the jaw jowls and gobbler neck that come with aging. My outlook on life is more positive and I react more positively even if something negative is happening around me. Over time, I know that eating a raw foods diet will help me live a long, healthy and productive life without all of the ailments I had while eating a standard American diet.

If you think eating a raw diet is time-consuming, inconvenient or even too tedious, I would like you to compare that little bit of additional effort to the experience of being on lifelong medications, or even dying, from the results of cancer or some other degenerative condition. Personally, I'd rather spend two days each month making delicious raw tortilla chips, drying fruit or preparing other foods than spend weeks, months or years in a hospital bed unable to do anything but wait to die.

I guess I don't need to tell you that I plan to make this a long-term lifestyle. Eating raw, along with body movement and meditation, is the way for me and there is no turning back. I've already cleared out my kitchen cupboards and have replaced everything. This is a lifetime commitment and I love it!

Sarah Chimblo, 35

Jenks, Oklahoma

As a mother of two and a teacher, I know the importance of eating raw foods for health. After the birth of my second child, I noticed that the last 15 pounds of pregnancy weight wasn't coming off as easily as it had the first time, eight years ago. So I started researching healthier food habits and came across the raw food lifestyle via Penni's blog, which was recommended by my sister-in-law. I decided to try the Raw Food Cleanse as a way to get my eating under control and to rethink how and what I was eating.

I did the three-day cleanse to begin with and experienced some of the symptoms of detox. I had the chills, a little more acne than usual and a runny nose. Those symptoms subsided as I continued eating raw after the cleanse. For one week during the experiment, I really focused on eating totally raw, and I exercised. Within that week I lost six pounds. That was a dress-size for me. I noticed that my post-baby clothes from a year ago are getting loose on me. I've gone from about 25 percent to 60–70 percent raw during the last 11 weeks.

What I've learned through this process:

Be prepared. If you are a parent, you'll need to plan your meals and how you can best incorporate your foods with the family meals.

Be kind to yourself. Some days all I could do was eat fruit and veggies as snacks, but then again, refer to the previous tip.

Smoothies are an easy alternative when you're on the go. They're great as a meal replacement for breakfast or lunch.

Green Smoothies are great for digestion. A simple combination of spinach, cucumber and apples has so many good nutrients.

When I eat more raw foods, my body just feels better on less food.

Participating in the Raw Food Cleanse has made me look more closely at the food I give my family. It has prompted research and led me to read many books about the food industry and how eating raw, unprocessed food really is best for my family. My goals in the future are to continue adding more fruits/veggies to my family's diet, curb the snacking that comes from the teacher's lounge and encourage others to eat real food.

Dianne, 50

Gig Harbor, Washington

Dianne was already rocking a high-raw-food diet before she started the Raw Food Cleanse, but during the 11 weeks she lost weight and noticed that her skin began to clear. People even started commenting on the weight loss in her face and the disappearance of her wrinkles. She also shared that her sleep patterns were improved, and that she required fewer hours of sleep per night to feel rested. She is totally on board with this lifestyle and plans to continue to eat a high-raw diet moving forward.

Marcy Lisboa, 39
Brooklyn, New York

Starting this experiment really made me look at myself more than at food. The detox we worked on hit home in more ways than one. It made me realize that my weight issues are about so much more than just what I was putting into my mouth. I have been controlling my feelings by stuffing food down. That realization was my biggest reward of this experiment and I'm so grateful for it.

I learned that the past is in the past and that I am more than just a number on a scale. The scale will no longer be the measure of who I am as a person. I now have a more positive self-image and I view this is as just the beginning for me. Weight management is just a small part of what I received from this experiment. I now have a sense that I can be successful in anything I seek to do. Look for my "full story" in Penni's sequel to this book—I am just starting to emerge from my cocoon!

Robin Abbott, 47
Little Rock, Arkansas

I first learned about raw foods, juicing and smoothies last year when I read *Health Bliss,* by Susan Smith Jones, which introduced the concept of the raw food lifestyle. It piqued my interest and I kept thinking and thinking about it. I did more research on the internet, and I went to the library and checked out Harvey Diamond's latest book (Harvey wrote *Fit For Life* in the '80s). I discovered Angela Stokes on the internet and downloaded her book, *Raw Emotions*. I began watching her and Matt Monarch on YouTube. That's where I ran across their interview with Penni the last weekend in May.

When I looked at Penni's site, she had posted an invitation to join in the Raw Food Cleanse Experiment. The timing was spot-on as the program would be starting in the next day or so. I thought about it for a short time and told my husband I wanted to do it. I told him it would take a lot of my time and energy, but I needed to do it. He was supportive, so I signed up.

I had gotten up to 180 pounds last year and had lost 14 pounds January through March of this year by eating whole cooked foods and exercising, but my weight loss had stalled. I went back to my standard American diet again in March and quit working out as my energy went down. The vicious cycle had begun again. On June 1, when this experiment began, I weighed in at 167, so I was really ready for a change!

Even though the changes were difficult at first, it took only a week for positive transformations to start occurring. I began feeling better and not minding the body movement or missing cooked food. After about a week, the physical food cravings subsided. I began saying positive affirmations when I was walking outside, on the treadmill, or driving. My favorite affirmation is, "I maintain optimum health and a slim, sexy body through a diet of living and raw foods, sunshine and exercise." I believe that a change in mindset has had as much to do with my transformation as the raw foods and exercise. Everything seemed to be completely intertwined.

Throughout this experiment, my diet mainly consisted of fresh fruit in the mornings, a Green

Smoothie in the late morning or at lunch, or leftovers from a raw food dinner at lunch. I would enjoy a Green Juice mid-afternoon and then have a raw food dinner an hour or so later. I enjoyed trying several of the Life Cleanse recipes along with others I found on the internet or in raw food books. Without a dehydrator or high-speed blender, I had to keep things as simple as possible.

I read in Tonya Zavasta's book *Beautiful on Raw* that transitioning to a raw food lifestyle is similar to immigrating to another country. There are many cultural activities that must be left behind. There are new friends to be made and new tastes to acquire. I still miss the ease of grabbing a quick processed meal, or going out to dinner and being waited on after a long day. But nothing compares with the improvement in health, physically, mentally and spiritually, that I have gained. I've gone from being an overweight, sluggish, perimenopausal emotional ping-pong ball with bad skin and high cholesterol, to a healthy, fit, happy and vibrant woman. Within 11 weeks I lost 23 pounds and I feel like I have my life back! I plan to maintain a high raw lifestyle for the rest of my life. I don't see any way of maintaining optimum health without eating a very high percentage of living foods, so I do plan to continue learning to prepare more raw recipes, and to get more involved in the raw food lifestyle.

Janine Gibbons, 49
Evergreen, Colorado

Janine went from 20 to 80 percent raw and lost eight pounds during the Raw Food Cleanse. Her boyfriend noticed that she was looking slimmer, which she found really encouraging, and her energy level was much improved. Eating a high-raw-food diet is now a lifelong choice as she continues to approach her goal weight and improve her long-term health.

Name withheld by request

I began drinking alcohol on a somewhat regular basis about ten years ago. Although I gave up alcohol for Lent one year, prior to doing the Raw Food Cleanse I was drinking nearly every evening. Usually it was two or three glasses of wine, and then other times it was the whole bottle. When I would go out I'd indulge in two or three margaritas or Long Island Teas. I didn't give my "habit" too much concern since drinking hadn't interfered with my life to the point where I didn't meet responsibilities, and no one had ever confronted me about it. But down deep, it weighed on my mind. My brother passed away due in part to alcoholism, and both of my mother's grandfathers were alcoholics, bringing much shame to the family.

When I made the decision to join the Raw Food Cleanse research group, I knew alcohol would interfere with my results, but I was concerned that I couldn't give up my evening wine. A part of me wondered if I'd become an alcoholic. I decided to not make a big deal out of it and made the decision to just go ahead and try. There was something unique about this situation that allowed me to approach things in a relaxed way, although I did feel accountable to the program and the rest of the group. It was really the perfect situation; after all, it was just an experiment.

Once on a high raw foods diet, I never had physical cravings for alcohol. Giving it up was no more difficult than giving up the unhealthy diet I had been eating. I just toughed it out that first week and then I was completely fine. Although I never considered myself an alcoholic, I was a regular drinker. Eating a raw food diet cured my cravings for sweets, alcohol, bread and other SAD foods. Oh, and coffee, too. I didn't think this was possible! One simple thing I've done to help with cravings is drink mineral water, or even plain water with lemon or lime in a pretty wine glass. I think part of why I enjoy drinking is holding the pretty glass. Silly, I know, but it works. No doubt the change in diet and the elimination of my daily alcohol is the reason I lost so much weight in 11 weeks, including a six-and-a-half-inch loss around my belly!

Melinda Gill, 38

Coquitlam, British Columbia

I was already eating a pretty high-raw-foods diet when I joined the Raw Food Cleanse project. I saw this as an opportunity to turn up the volume and get serious about eating 100 percent raw for the duration of the experiment. Even though I already had experienced a marked improvement in my health since going raw, bumping it up to 100 percent brought these exciting changes: clearer skin with a definite glow, better mood, weight loss of over 14 pounds, much better elimination, able to deal with adversity better, and less aches and pains in general. My energy levels are great and I need much less sleep. I just do so much better at 100 percent raw. My hormones and monthly cycle have balanced out, which is awesome, especially since I will be trying to conceive within the next couple of months. Wouldn't it be neat to have a Raw Food Cleanse baby?!

Wendy Campbell, 46
Oklahoma City, Oklahoma

I struggled with my weight for years due to hypothyroidism. After four years of thyroid medication adjustments and dieting (Weight Watchers, Atkins and South Beach) I finally lost 112 pounds, placing me at my goal weight of 128 pounds. I was at this weight for only three months when I got a diagnosis of adrenal failure and was put on cortisone for life. I was told I would die without it. I immediately started gaining weight (this was in 2004). Then I got very ill in 2008 with drug-induced Cushing's Syndrome (the opposite of adrenal failure). I weaned myself off the cortisone very slowly. It took five months, and I did not die. My most recent doctor believes I was misdiagnosed because the proper tests were never done. I've now been off cortisone for four months and am still healing from Cushing's Syndrome.

I also have gastroparesis (gut paralysis). My entire digestive tract was not working properly from my stomach to my colon. My food would not digest and I had severe constipation. I had daily nausea and vomited several times a week. I had reflux 24/7. When what little I ate did stay down, the food would stay in my stomach for days and ferment. The bloating was unbearable. My colon barely worked and I had to take a gallon of Miralax once a week to get a weekly BM. I lost 50 pounds and suffered from malabsorption and anemia. I tried many medications, but none worked. I was told that my last resort would be a total liquid diet; if that were to fail I would need colon surgery. Meat, fat and fiber are the hardest things for me to digest so the medically suggested "gastroparesis diet" is highly refined starches with very low fiber. Fiber can cause bezoars—fiber balls akin to the hairballs cats get—that have to be surgically removed.

Over the last year I tried the GP diet, vegetarianism and veganism. I was sicker than ever, vomiting more and had no choice but to switch to a completely liquid diet in April 2009. I started with smoothies. I knew to get as much nourishment as I could I needed whole foods. I also bought a juicer. This was the beginning of raw for me. Within a week I no longer experienced nausea, vomiting or bloating and I didn't need any more medications to have a BM. I now go up to three times a day; apparently fiber is not an issue if it's raw.

After a few weeks on smoothies I tried small amounts of fruits and did not get sick. Then I tried a few nuts and did not get sick. I was very afraid of veggies because they had made me so sick in the past. It took about a month for me to try some zucchini with a little marinara. I did not get sick.

It's a total miracle that my stomach works as long as I stay raw. It's a miracle that I've lost 15 pounds in 17 days while still healing from Cushing's. I'd like to lose more weight and would love to get off as many of the drugs as I can. I also want people to know that the raw food diet can be a miracle, and it can happen so fast!

Since participating in the Raw Food Cleanse, I've been consuming more juices, smoothies and raw food, and I am so much better. I have been able to stop taking my diabetes meds, as my blood sugar is staying well within the normal range, and I have also stopped taking Celexa for depression. I have become interested in yoga, taking raja and hatha yoga classes, and started jogging. I have never heard of anyone healing themselves of gastroparesis *and* diabetes through a raw diet. As you can imagine, I now want to spread this message of healing and help everyone I can.

Ann Kaye, 49
Baltimore, Maryland

Even though I was a vegetarian for 28 years, my diet was mainly junk-food vegetarian and only about 20 percent fruits and vegetables. My acidic diet, coupled with the poisonous stress hormones from a major depressive episode/spiritual crisis, were the breeding ground that later led to my breast cancer diagnosis. At that time I instinctively knew I had to clean up my diet. I became a vegan and immersed myself in studies of nutrition and cancer. After much research, I am convinced that the benefits of a diet consisting of pure, fresh, unprocessed foods are superlative and without question the right path for my continued good health!

Ellen Morrison, 42
Honolulu, Hawaii

I have realized the benefit of raw for years now but had not yet embraced the lifestyle completely. Prior to this experiment, I was eating mostly vegetarian and trying to have at least one salad per day. The biggest change that I made during the cleanse was to have a green smoothie every morning religiously. I also did yoga every single night so I was eating my heavier meal during the day and a much lighter meal in the evening.

I feel like all I've learned has helped me to change on so many levels. That is why I am certain that I will lose the weight and keep it off this time. I feel like I am becoming a new person. But really I am just coming into a fuller expression of my truest, best self.

Samantha Gibbs, 34
Dearborn Heights, Michigan

I love raw food and what it has done for me. It has opened up a whole new way of living. I am 34 years old and for about 32 of those years I lived on junk food. I used to joke that I should become a vegetarian but I hated vegetables! I have always hated any and all healthy food. I could and would try to live on cookies (preferably the dough), salt bagels dipped in blue cheese dressing, pretzels, cake, cheese, bread, basically anything carb-ish. The only vegetable I would touch was cucumber and that was only with iodized salt and dressing. I probably ate one piece of fruit a month. When I had to, I would eat a meal, but I preferred to eat junk instead.

I started learning about raw foods when my husband became sick with ulcerative colitis. I learned even more when my son was born with food allergies to dairy, nuts and eggs. I honestly had no idea what to feed him. I started eating more fruits and trying to add veggies in when I could, and it was then that I really started trying to change the way I fed my whole family.

I came up with a plan to try to go 100 percent raw and blog about it. My start date was to be June 1. It was then that I learned about the Raw Food Cleanse research project and decided it would be the perfect support so I signed up. I got through the first 30 days 100 percent raw and blogged every day about what I ate: calories, fat, etc. After the 30 days, I unfortunately started letting things slip back in—like tortilla chips or popcorn. In the eyes of the average American I was still eating healthy, but I could instantly tell a difference in the way I felt and looked. I have since struggled to stay 100 percent raw, which is a personal goal of mine, but I did lose 12 pounds during the course of the 11 weeks.

This experience has made me realize how passionate I am about raw food and sharing it with others. I've just finished creating a raw foods website/business; I am writing an e-book and will be holding classes and demos showing moms how to feed their children healthy, fresh foods. I would even love to have classes geared for children where I show them some yummy recipes to make! I am by no means a raw food expert but I really want to share everything I have learned with other moms. I hope that I can make a big impact where I live!

Amy Reutter, 40
Tulsa, Oklahoma

I feel so much better if I am eating exclusively raw. My moods are better. My cravings for the standard American diet eventually go away. I have also found that transitioning to eating raw starts in my mind and spirit. It's a decision I make when I wake up in the morning. Even though I don't naturally crave Green Smoothies at first, I have to just *decide* to drink them for a period of time. Eventually my body takes over and starts to crave the good stuff on its own, and my spirit keeps everything in check. When I get to this point, social situations where cooked food is abundant aren't as hard.

During the 11-week experiment, I noticed my mood and emotions would get heavy when I ate cooked foods. The irritability, depression, PMS, you name it, would come right back. I've learned that I feel sooo much better on raw! This is a lifestyle that I will continue with from now on.

Kimberly Graham, 45
Indianola, Iowa

In many ways, this experience has been a rebirth for me. I can't fully articulate the alchemy of it all, but things came together during the Raw Food Cleanse that have never coalesced this way before. I feel better able to nourish myself—to choose not only healthy but delicious foods that feed my body, soul, heart and spirit.

Many people think we must be eating cardboard if we are eating "healthy" and "raw." Of course I know this couldn't be further from the truth. I've always loved real, whole foods best, and since I'm a food snob, if something doesn't taste yummy, I won't eat it. So believe me when I say I have not been eating cardboard! In addition to fabulous raw breakfast, lunch and dinner meals, I've learned to make raw goodies that satisfy my cravings for chocolate, ice cream, and even the fattier foods. They are made with whole, raw ingredients and I use low-glycemic sweeteners and only the good fats our bodies need.

I plan to eat a high-raw-food diet moving forward. I always enjoyed eating fruits and vegetables, but usually got tired of them because I didn't have varied and delicious ways to prepare them. Now I do. I view this more as a lifestyle choice than just about the weight loss. Of course I'm thrilled to have released 18 pounds, but the overall health impact is more important to me in the long term.

Linda Ann Recupito, 54
Crete, Illinois

I'm not sure where I was headed when I began the Raw Food Cleanse. I've always eaten well—sometimes too well. Now I truly look at the health value of the food that I eat. It is amazing that changing your intake of living foods can have such a positive effect on your body, mind and spirit. I have been told my eyes are bluer. Can you imagine that the food you eat can affect your eye color? Green Smoothies are by far my breakfast of choice. You cannot get a healthier or easier breakfast, in my opinion. I crave greens and I can tell when I am not getting enough; my body will start to crave foods that are not good for me. It was really beneficial to learn that upping my intake of leafy greens helps to manage cravings.

The improvement in my energy level was so dramatic. It was enough to get me up out of bed every morning at 4:30 a.m., ready to go to the gym. I seriously haven't had this much energy in years. I would recommend trying this way of eating to anyone. It was an amazing journey for my body, mind and spirit. I feel a sense of gratitude for the opportunity because I have learned so much. It has changed my life.

Heather Wolf, 32
Eugene, Oregon

The Raw Food Cleanse was just a starting place for me. It was a totally positive experience and I learned so much. This was my first time trying to do something like this, and I believe it will become easier and I'll be even more successful as time goes on. I know the weight will start coming off as I press on no matter what. I doubled my raw food intake during the 11 weeks, which was a big deal for me.

Although I wish I could have done better, I absolutely know that I am so much better off now than before I started. This is how I desire to eat and the way I want to feed myself and my family. I know in my heart that this is such a healthy lifestyle for the long term.

Suezee, 45
Naples, Florida

Raw foods have completely changed my life. For the first time ever, I feel connected to God. I went from 50 percent to nearly 100 percent raw in 11 weeks and lost 11 pounds. I have much more energy now. I started walking—I need to get out and walk, and this program got me going to the park and walking. This was huge! It was always on my to-do list, but I hadn't really done it until I got started with the Raw Food Cleanse.

My periods have also become normal, just like they were when I was young. HUGE!

I have more love, more energy, more compassion—I am peaceful. Life is good. After experiencing how I feel on raw, it would be very hard to go back to cooked food. I want to stay raw for my weight and health, but also for the way raw makes me feel. Sometimes I feel bliss. Cooked never did that for me.

Lowanna Hugall, 36
Perth, Australia

I knew Penni from the online community at RawFu. Even though I had already started with a raw food diet months earlier, I decided to support her research project and sign up to be a guinea pig. The main change I noticed during the Raw Food Cleanse Experiment was an improvement in my mental clarity, which has brought more emotional balance. I also started incorporating an exercise program into my routine, and

I pleasantly dropped an additional 23 pounds during the 11-week experiment.

Raw food has turned my life around 180 degrees. I can love more, appreciate others more and enjoy a better connection to myself and my spirit. I attribute all of this to being more nourished, which is what a raw lifestyle has offered me. My body is now no longer fighting to be fed. Today, instead of eating to cover up what's not working in my life, my focus is on giving my body raw meals that are of the highest nutrition possible. Today I honor and nurture myself. The food addictions that ran my life and took me away from living are a thing of the past. My body no longer demands and suffers with cravings, as now I am listening to what I really need. The struggle of malnutrition is over and all that is left is living and loving my life to the fullest each day.

Lowanna's achievements are truly amazing, and she was such an inspiration to the group. Choosing to simply eat raw consistently since the end of 2008 has meant she has lost well over 100 pounds. Today Lowanna continues her raw lifestyle and is a living advocate of the benefits a raw life can offer. You can follow her progress and watch her teaching on YouTube (see "Recommended YouTube Channels" in the Resources section).]

Karla Davis, 50
Jefferson, Georgia

I went from 20 percent to 90 percent raw during the course of the Raw Food Cleanse. My goal with raw foods was to maintain weight loss without having to count calories. As I began incorporating more raw foods into my diet, I found a wonderful side benefit. My rosacea, which I've had since I was in my early twenties, is gone. If I stay healthy and raw, it stays gone! So all that has been said about rosacea being affected by foods is true, but it's not just chocolate or caffeine, because I've cut those out before. Living foods have been the only thing that has kept my skin even-toned!

Deb LaTonzea, 42
Columbus, Ohio

Although I have not lost a huge amount of weight, my relationship with food has changed. I now recognize when I am truly hungry or eating emotionally. I was also dealing with a major health issue during this time, and everything I've learned in this program has helped me to understand that there is healing energy in the enzymes of live food.

I was able to double my raw food intake during these 11 weeks, and my goal is to stay around 75 percent raw. I am choosing this as a lifestyle—it's not about the weight. I love myself now and I would love me even if I didn't weigh less. I just want to be healthy in my mind, body and soul.

Kali Amato, 48
Lorain, Ohio

When I juice, drink Green Smoothies and eat fruits/veggies and salads, I feel awesome. I feel so connected to Spirit and feel the energy flowing through me and with me. When I eat foods like nuts, seeds, coconuts and avocados, I feel heavy and disconnected, so I'm learning to be mindful of that, reminding myself that more than one serving of those foods lowers my energy and seems to contribute to addictive eating patterns. This cleanse has helped me to be more aware of following my body's signals to discover what I need to do for optimal health, not listening to others' opinions of what is best. I have to be my own guru. I lost over 11 pounds, and I see this as part of my lifestyle for the long term.

Sally Jane, 41
Angola, Indiana

Over the past few weeks, I've really noticed changes when I eat a higher raw diet. My mental clarity is improved, I feel truly optimistic and suddenly have a desire for exercise! I've started walking, which is a substantial accomplishment for me. I see the Raw Food Cleanse as a way to achieve your weight-loss goals as well as a long-term lifestyle choice for optimum health!

Susan Bradbury, 47
Iron Mountain, Michigan

Last Labor Day weekend, I felt like I was having a heart attack. I had major pains down my entire left side for three days. Being stubborn, I waited to go to the doctor until I felt I could drive myself. My blood pressure was off the charts at 220/120 . . . strokeville! I was hospitalized for three days, but afterward I didn't fill the prescriptions: I decided to change my lifestyle instead. When I was finally *forced* to deal with these intense health issues, I chose a change of lifestyle over popping pills for symptoms. I knew the prescriptions would only be a Band-Aid.

It was then that I started with raw foods. During the first three months, I lost 28 pounds, and that was with a broken foot that I couldn't even stand on. I began as a very tight size 16 and today I'm a size 8. I am healthier than I have ever been! I just want to continue to shape up and not settle for "good enough."

This is definitely a long-term lifestyle choice for me. I will never go back to the low-energy, overweight, brain-fog, SAD (standard American diet) lifestyle ever again! Eating this way is easy, fun and delicious. You cannot pry my green smoothie out of my hand, or any of my raw food goodies like kale chips and raw chocolate cheesecake! This experiment has taken me to the next level in my life. The timing was perfect; it's been life-changing, and for that I will be eternally grateful. I have made many friends who will continue walking with me along this raw journey—wonderful friends for life!

Jeannette Marchand, 53
Westhampton, Massachusetts

Since I went raw and gave up coffee, my bursitis is gone and my eczema disappeared. My once-dry skin is now soft and supple, there's no more keratosis pilaris on my arms and legs, and my joints don't hurt. Lines on my face have diminished, revealing younger-looking skin. I've even noticed some regrowth of the outer third of my eyebrows. Not only is my breath sweeter, I've also noticed that body odor is mostly nonexistent. My breasts do not swell from eating or drinking certain foods anymore and my long-standing acid reflux is gone.

Because I can move faster without joint pain, I've added hula-hooping classes two times a week and I've started walking a half mile every other day. Although I have ADD, I am noticeably more calm and not as easily flustered. I am postmenopausal but have noticed a return of hot flashes since going raw. Does that mean I'm getting younger?!

During the Raw Food Cleanse, I've come to realize that I don't have to be 100 percent raw to live a really healthy life. It's okay to have some steamed veggies or pickled beets if that is what is available. I do try to stick with the veggies and fruits when making non-raw choices, however.

Even though I started this raw food journey to lose weight, the health benefits have been so considerable that I plan to make this a permanent way of life. I have slowly incorporated raw foods into my family's diet and am already starting to see benefits in their health as well. I don't expect them to go totally raw, but they'll certainly be making healthier choices in their non-raw foods.

Most of us who did the experiment found that we needed less food then we were eating before. I am sure it is because we are finally getting the nutrients from the foods we are eating. Even though I read a lot, being part of the group added to the overall experience in many ways. I also liked the fact that not being 100 percent raw was okay on the Raw Food Cleanse and that the 100-percent-raw police would not get on your case. This will be a lifestyle choice for me from here on out.

Jean had started eating raw food several months before she joined the Raw Food Cleanse Experiment, but she really kicked her personal program into high gear, dropping 22 pounds of her 46-pound total weight loss to the curb during the 11-week research program.

Eva Gapski, 24
Wellington, New Zealand

Since I began the Raw Food Cleanse, my mental clarity has improved significantly. I'm a full-time student and work part time so often I leave the house around 7:30 a.m. and return at 5:30 p.m. or later then have to study well into the evenings. With raw foods, I can just keep going until I decide it's time for bed. I have no afternoon slumps, my eyes don't fall shut anymore in boring meetings, and I seem to have endless energy.

I've noticed some other nice changes, too. My period has become shorter and lighter—no more cramps at all— and emotionally, I'm a lot happier, cheerful and positive. People say my happiness is infectious and they like my attitude, my outlook on life and my caring nature. Friends and acquaintances say I look radiant, healthy and happy. Some people focus on the weight loss and get worried, but often they're just jealous. I feel a lot more comfortable with my body and my weight now.

I will maintain my 90–100 percent raw diet for the rest of my life. The 10 percent is an allowance for going out to dinner with my boyfriend, for traveling, etc. This is definitely part of my life now, not just a means to an end.

Lisa Hudson, 43
Columbia, Tennessee

I ate anything I wanted until 13 years ago when we moved to Tennessee. I took an office job after being a housewife forever, and within six months I packed on 65 pounds. Over the last 12 years, I've tried to lose weight with so many diets I can't even count anymore. Each time I would do really well for two or three weeks and then end up bingeing on the weekend, gaining it all back plus some on top of that. I beat myself up each time.

During this time, I also had my last child. I was so unhappy with my life and couldn't understand why I couldn't beat this thing. My skin was really bad and I tried everything I knew to correct that, but with no luck. I had GERD (acid reflux) and was drinking water with baking soda every night to go to sleep. For about three years I would vomit in the night because of the GERD.

One day when I was watching YouTube, I came across a video that said "RAW VEGAN" and I watched it. That day I probably watched 35 to 40 videos and found so many new and helpful websites. I went raw that day, haven't turned back and never will. I've even changed what I want to do with the rest of my life. I want to open a raw food restaurant and store in my town. I have lost a total of 35 pounds since I went raw and 15 during the Raw Food Cleanse Experiment. I truly feel amazing. This has become a life-transforming way of life for me, with no turning back. I can't shut up about raw foods.

Leigh, 55, and Megan, 31 (mother and daughter)

Tulsa, Oklahoma

Leigh says:

Honestly, I just feel better when I eat raw. Food seems to taste better and cleaner. For instance, I've noticed that I can eat a potato and I don't need to pile a bunch of other stuff on it to taste good. I actually enjoy the taste of the potato in and of itself. I notice the simple goodness of real food now. I find that I am much less a meat-based person now that I eat a high-raw-foods diet. I just don't crave it anymore.

I love fresh juice and fresh smoothies. "Clean" is the word that keeps coming to me. I was diagnosed with a fairly rare form of cancer before upping my raw food intake. Once I realized what I was dealing with, I became very serious about what I was putting into my mouth and my overall lifestyle choices. I was able to tolerate hideous, horrible chemo—chemo that is not FDA-approved outside of Houston Medical Center— plus four surgeries, like a 25-year-old (those were the doctor's very words).

I've not only survived but am continuing to survive this cancer. I attribute this in large part to my diet. During chemo, when I could not eat much of anything, I could always eat raw and I craved fresh juices, particularly orange and carrot/apple juice. Even at my most nauseated I could always drink fresh, raw juices. Sometimes that was all I could keep down.

Now I've started running with my daughter, Megan, who joined me in the Raw Food Cleanse Experiment. We've each lost well over 10 pounds and we feel great. There's no doubt that this is a lifestyle we'll both continue well into the future.

And from Megan:

My mother was diagnosed with a rare cancer in my adult years. She wasn't given good odds of survival, so I was determined to help her find what would make her thrive. As a family we have made more of a conscious effort to eat our way to health through real food. My mother has recovered very well and has beaten the odds. I truly believe our bodies were made to heal themselves as long as we don't get in the way. We were designed to eat the fruits of the land, and if people would go back to the basics they would find that they are in control of their own health. Just because we continually get older, it doesn't mean we have to feel that way.

Melodie Bertoli, 51
Antioch, Tennessee

I met Melodie on RawFu and we've been internet buddies for quite a while now. Like many others, Melodie has struggled with her diet, so I was excited that she signed up to be one of our research participants. One of her biggest motivations in changing her diet for good has been observing her mother's illness and dependency on prescription drugs. She wants a better life for herself.

I'm so proud of Melodie. She kicked 14 unwanted pounds to the curb while doing the Raw Food Cleanse, and she learned to like Green Smoothies as long as she used spinach (she's not a big fan of kale!). She plans to make the raw food lifestyle her permanent approach to eating so she can experience the best health possible well into old age!

Margie, 46
Merriville, Indiana

When this experiment was first talked about, I couldn't wait to start. At first I was very committed, but then things in my personal life interrupted, which meant that I didn't eat 100 percent raw, which had been my goal. At times I would eat unhealthy things, but overall I did pretty well. I do feel much better than I did 11 weeks ago.

Some benefits of doing the Raw Food Cleanse: I sleep so much better. My hot flashes disappeared. Pain from my trigger thumb is gone. My hair stopped falling out and seems much fuller. I feel a new sense of calm, almost like an inner peace. Although this feeling isn't constant, it is certainly there. Sometimes I'm aware that there is a feeling flowing through me like I am oozing love out of every pore. Maybe this is an endorphin high. It's a good feeling!

I'm leaning toward a more simple way of life, and I feel that a raw food diet is the simplest way to eat. This lifestyle is also one that leaves a smaller footprint. Now that I buy items with "natural" packaging, I have very little trash. I love having a blended smoothie for a meal. It's the easiest way to get a lot of fruits and vegetables in, especially the greens. Juicing is another way to get nutrients, but without the fiber. I don't like it as much as smoothies, but I did juice an entire watermelon yesterday and it was amazing—*really* refreshing.

Not only am I using raw food for weight loss, I'm also using it for disease prevention. I'm at the age where things can really begin to fall apart, and I've been pretty lucky so far. You can have all the money in the world, but without your health, you have nothing. This way of eating is paving the road for a long, healthy life ahead!

Delaney Berrini, 33
Minneapolis, Minnesota

Even though I had followed a raw food diet before finding the Raw Food Cleanse opportunity, I feel like I was able to go raw and stay high raw this time because of my discipline with green juices. No matter what, every morning, I juiced. With the greens flowing through me, I had no cravings for anything that wasn't good for my body or part of my journey. Plus the juicing allowed me to eat fewer meals and helped my digestion because I wasn't snacking all day. Normally, I eat all day. Juicing is king!

During the 11 weeks, I was able to let go of dates and nuts and heavy raw foods (including coconut butter) that I had struggled with in the past. I love my body now and love waking up and going to the gym. I feel clean! For two months of this program I ate 80 percent fruit and 20 percent vegetables. I think this served its purpose, so now I'm back to steaming and baking yams occasionally for dinner. I'm not stressing so much about my "rawness" like I did in the past. I realize that I may eat more or less fat or more or less fruit along my journey but I will stay high raw. The key is not becoming too dogmatic. I have to monitor and see how my body reacts as I switch things in and out of my diet. I cannot follow raw "gurus" and make their diets mine. I have to figure it out for myself. This is a big lesson I learned.

I've continued to release weight, 17 pounds altogether, and even though I'm slender now, I feel that my body is still surprising me with new healthful discoveries. One of the best discoveries for me was that I can still build muscle without eating meat. I used to be into a high protein diet (in my twenties) and dated men who insisted I had to eat meat to build muscle. I saw an ex-boyfriend over the weekend. I was carrying a box, and he commented on my muscled arms. I said, "Yeah. Nice, huh?" He said, "Even without protein. . . ." Fruits and veggies *have* protein!

Ronna Wheeler, 44
Richmond, Vermont

I have been on lots and lots of diets in the past 20 years. I always felt fat, even when I wasn't. I lost 20 pounds on Weight Watchers about 10 years ago, and gained it all back and then some when I stopped "counting points." I lost 20 pounds while trekking around Nepal and gained it back when I got back to the

U.S. I gained 40 pounds with each pregnancy and only lost about half of that.

This is honestly the first time I've looked at my eating habits as a lifestyle choice, and not as a diet. The Raw Food Cleanse is totally different. I want to be healthy, feel good, look good, and if the pounds come off, even better. I love learning about eating raw, juice feasting, supplements, detox, etc. There is so much info out there and it can be challenging to sort through it all, but the information in this program helps bring it all together. I've been able to go from 25 percent to 75 percent raw during the past 11 weeks!

To achieve my weight-loss goals and for my overall good health, I choose this as a long-term lifestyle. I had gestational diabetes with both of my children and am at high risk for developing full-blown diabetes. Right now my fasting blood sugars hover around 100, which is borderline, and this gives me added motivation to stay raw. I want to be healthy for my children (now three and five years old) and I want the energy to keep up with them. Raw food is definitely the way to go for life!

Caroline, 66, and Heather, 42 (mother and daughter)

Apple Valley, California

Caroline grew up eating raw foods and has been interested in a healthy natural diet her whole life. During the 11-week Raw Food Cleanse Experiment, she went from a diet of 60 percent to over 90 percent raw. Caroline feels that eating this way is in part an act of obedience to God, as she is better able to hear His voice when she is in a fasted state, ready for service. She happily lost over eight pounds during this time and will continue to incorporate a high level of raw foods into her daily diet. Caroline held a precious presence within the group, and her quiet prayers were felt by many.

Caroline's daughter, Heather, also participated in the Raw Food Cleanse Experiment. Here's what she had to say about the experience:

In November of 2008, I was searching for weight-loss stories on YouTube. One in particular that I found was Angela Stokes-Monarch. I was really amazed at how beautiful she was after her dramatic weight loss. She looked healthy, hydrated and happy. I was also encouraged, thinking, *"She was fatter than me!* I only need to lose 60 pounds. I love vegetables, fruits, nuts and seeds; I like raw food. . . . I can do this!" So on November 15, 2008, I started my raw food journey. Beginning weight: 206 pounds.

YouTube became my raw food information headquarters. I subscribed to around 50 raw food channels and received at least two or three new videos a day. This is where I found the lovely Penni Shelton. A very pretty blue-eyed redhead like myself, Penni was already successful on raw food. She gave me a vision.

I quickly learned that the key to success with this way of eating was preparation. I would cut up salad for three hours (12 heads of romaine lettuce with all the fixings) about every four days. Package it up in Ziploc bags. My refrigerator was immediately turned into my new fast food drive-thru. I would eat seasonal fruit. When I first started, apples were in season and they tasted amazing. I would eat three or four apples a day. When I started green smoothies, I noticed my cravings went away. This became the way I could get enough nutrients into my body. I now consume two or three bunches of kale a day in the form of smoothies.

The first week I lost 10 pounds. I was stoked. In 40 days I lost 24 pounds. By February 15, I had lost 45 pounds—down to 161 pounds. The best part about it was that I was eating *all the time*.

After my weight loss of 45 pounds, I started trying out more raw recipes, desserts, eating more avocado, etc., and gained back five pounds. I have successfully maintained my weight loss and lifestyle for five months now. I have never felt better. I believe I will maintain this way of eating for the rest of my life and look forward to reaching my goal weight of 146 pounds by my one-year Raw Anniversary.

Stasi Torrez, 45
Granbury, Texas

Stasi had some pretty substantial life changes during the 11 weeks of the Raw Food Cleanse Experiment. Even without her full focus, she was able to drop almost 10 pounds and go from eating 30 percent raw to about 60 percent in her daily diet. Losing two inches in her waist and two and a half inches in her hips is encouragement enough to keep her plugged into this as a long-term lifestyle choice as she continues to work toward her ultimate weight-loss goals.

Jenneca McCarter, 21
Broken Arrow, Oklahoma

I've only been following a high-raw lifestyle for a couple of months, but I can already tell my body is slowly healing from a lifetime of stomach issues. It's amazing to not have to take any antacids or prescriptions on a regular basis! I avoid taking conventional medications when at all possible, so this is an awesome accomplishment. The raw foods are also slowly helping me deal with body image issues I have had for a long time. Due to my stomach problems, I was always overweight and bloated as a young girl and I took a lot of teasing because of it. As I've gotten older, I've begun to think about what I'm eating and how I'm moving my body, and I have started slowly losing weight over a few years.

Through this experiment I have come to realize that the way I had been viewing my body wasn't healthy. Raw foods have provided a calming effect for me at this point. I know that what I am putting into my body is healthy, and that with time and increased exercise, I will be able to do whatever I want because I will be able to achieve the fitness level I am striving for. This lifestyle is slowly allowing me to let go. I don't have to think about how I look 24/7 because I know I will ultimately reach my goal.

I plan to continue increasing the amounts of raw foods I am eating until I can get close to maintaining a 100 percent lifestyle. I want to use raw foods as a tool to assist me with weight loss, but my main focus is using raw foods as a way to heal my body from IBS/acid reflux issues once and for all. Eating raw is a way to heal my body, mind and spirit while staying healthy and increasing my physical fitness. I see this as a long-term lifestyle choice.

MaKenzie Maxwell, 42
Gaithersburg, Maryland

Since doing the raw thing I've been better able to juggle multiple tasks and I've become better organized. This is so important to note because I have ADHD (attention deficit hyperactivity disorder) for which I cannot take "traditional meds" due to my heart condition. I've also noticed that I get by with a lot less sleep than before. I know I can lose weight through a raw foods lifestyle. Perhaps I can also reverse some of the damage to my heart caused by eating the junk that got me into having so many physical problems to begin with. It's my health issues that make this journey so very important to me. My health may depend on whether I can sustain a raw lifestyle.

I'm looking forward to equipping my kitchen and embracing what it takes to be a success at this for the long haul!

Tracey Crider, 52
Biloxi, Mississippi

When I am eating raw, I lose weight, have more energy, need less sleep, have fewer menopausal symptoms, headaches and mood swings, and the achiness in my legs disappears. My cravings for sweet food and junk food disappear almost completely and my appetite drops dramatically—to the point that I almost have to *make* myself eat. I become regular with my "poop schedule," am less irritable, sleep more soundly, think more clearly, save money, have more time because it's quicker to prepare food this way, and am generally healthier and happier.

Even though there have been a number of stressors in my life during the cleanse program, I really appreciate what I've learned and the people I've met. I will certainly continue on this path. I've even started a local raw food meet-up group in my area for additional support. I'm looking forward to achieving my weight-loss goals and staying with the lifestyle for weight and health maintenance.

Roxana Wolfe, 38
Galloway, Ohio

Having just finished the Raw Food Cleanse Experiment, I am more ready than ever to take control of my health. People have said they notice a certain glow about me, and I've lost some weight and an inch around my waist. Moving forward I plan to continue to eat more raw food and would like to be part of more raw challenges.

Eve Hamner, 62
Nevada City, California

I have been reading about and trying raw foods off and on for years. I've bought a lot of the books, looked at a lot of the raw websites, and even went to a raw event here in town when David Wolfe came, but it was only when I signed up for the Raw Food Cleanse that I actually buckled down and really embraced the lifestyle. Something about the approach made me feel safe. Actually, I think it was fate.

I was surfing the net one day when I came across Penni's name and I clicked on it. It happened to be a Sunday, May 31, the last day to sign up as a guinea pig for the Raw Food Cleanse Experiment. I debated—should I or not? Well, something in me said to do it, and I'm so glad that I did. I have lost 22 pounds so far and I'm still losing. I've learned so much, met wonderful like-minded people, and acquired some great tips and lots of recipes.

There is no doubt that I will definitely continue with a high-raw diet. I prefer being higher than 80 percent raw, both for weight loss and for a long-term lifestyle. As I move forward, I'll try more recipes (especially smoothie and juice recipes), use all my raw kitchen equipment, start dehydrating things, and be more of an example to other family members. I intend to educate myself more, keep up my raw daily journal (it helps me with accountability to myself), keep up with body movement and dry-brush massage and, of course, drink more water.

I am not 100 percent raw yet, but am still getting wonderful results. I'm calmer, happier, and have tons more energy; it feels like I am finally doing something right for myself. This is the longest that I have ever done almost all raw. I am so happy because I've realized that I CAN do this! I've even had the opportunity to say, "It must be the Green Smoothies!" several times to different people. I will be forever grateful for this program as it's been a life-changing process for me!

Dennis Clark, 45
Southern Alabama

Before Dennis tells you about his Raw Food Cleanse experience, I want to give you a bit of background on our "biggest loser." Dennis is not genetically obese; as a matter of fact, he used to be quite the athlete in high school, lettering in a few sports. He even served in the United States military for a few years, maintaining a buff, athletic build. His family of origin are all average-sized people. So, when Dennis signed up as one of my research guinea pigs, I wanted to know his story. How did Dennis end up topping the scales at nearly 550 pounds just two years ago?

From the very beginning, I was particularly fascinated with Dennis's positive can-do attitude, and even though he weighed in a few hundred pounds heavier than all the other participants, I knew there was something different, something very special about Dennis. In an early e-mail, Dennis shared details of his personal story, and we have talked via telephone many times since.

Dennis began to put on weight in his mid twenties. At that time he went through a very stressful marriage and separation, and it was then that he began to seek comfort in food. Once officially divorced, he gravitated toward fast, convenient food as a way of life and to pacify himself, especially late at night. As the years went by, Dennis kept getting larger.

Dennis's career afforded him the financial ability to eat out whenever he liked. Since he traveled a lot in his profession, he would enjoy dining out often, usually for all three meals, including a late-night drive-thru habit as a reward for working long, hard days. Food was his comfort, but over time his eating patterns and dramatic weight gain began to deeply concern his family and close friends.

Dennis shared that at one point he would drive to a local recycling facility in the middle of the night to secretly weigh himself on their one-ton commercial utility scale. This is actually how he found out that he was pushing 550 pounds. This was his first wake-up call, so he scheduled an appointment with a nearby doctor who performed gastric bypass surgery, thinking that would be his only hope.

After a three-hour seminar and a one-hour preliminary consultation with the doctor, Dennis learned that this doctor would not agree to do the surgery for insurance reasons. At this point, Dennis nearly lost all hope for ever living a normal life again. One precious detail that Dennis shared with me is that no matter what happened, his mother never gave up on him. She was always loving, encouraging and non-judgmental, even though he knew she was deeply concerned about his binge eating and weight.

A few more years passed and Dennis saved enough money for a newer procedure that was being offered in his area, Lap-Band surgery. He made the appointment once he had the funds together (nearly $20K) and eagerly went to talk with the doctor, ready to schedule the surgery. After spending a good amount of time on all the preliminaries, the doctor came in only to tell Dennis that the hospital wouldn't allow the surgery to be done on anyone over 400 pounds. Dejected once again, Dennis became hopeless.

To make matters worse, the downturn in the economy created a near standstill in Dennis's line of work. With the stock market crashing and the housing market nearly down the tubes, in January 2008 Dennis decided to move in with his mother and stepfather as a way to stay afloat in uncertain economic times. This move turned out to be a good situation, as his mother's cooking was relatively healthy and she even encouraged him to use his YMCA membership to get some much-needed exercise. Dennis's aunt gave him the book *God's Way* by George Malkmus, which planted the first seed in his mind of raw foods. Exercise and his mother's cooking helped Dennis lose about 40 pounds that year, which was encouraging, but hardly a dent in his massive frame.

In May of 2009, Dennis hit another low point. His mother had made a large meal one Sunday morning before going to church. The meal was one of Dennis's favorites—the main entrée was a big casserole dish of shepherd's pie. Normally Dennis would enjoy the Sunday meal with his parents after they returned home from church. This particular Sunday his parents decided to stay at church for a lunch event, and they told Dennis to go ahead and have lunch without them. By the time they arrived home, Dennis had devoured the entire meal, leaving not even a morsel for his family. His parents were startled and deeply concerned when they realized that he had eaten a meal large enough to serve at least six adults—in one sitting, all by himself. Dennis immediately felt rage, but he also realized things had spiraled out of control. The guilt and humiliation from this episode is what ultimately led him to the Raw Food Cleanse. There was no doubt in either of our minds that God ultimately orchestrated Dennis's finding my video calling for willing guinea pigs that afternoon.

I started the Raw Food Cleanse Experiment on June 1, 2009. I weighed in at 484.6 pounds, and I was extremely unhappy (even if I didn't admit it). After just two weeks on the program, I had lost 24 pounds, and man, were my eyes suddenly wide open to a whole new world! For the next nine weeks I continued to lose weight at an average rate of 4 pounds a week. I even did a three-day juice cleanse, which totally cleaned out my system and gave me tons of energy. When I made salads I would use anywhere from 13 to 20 different ingredients; the more, the better! My world opened up to chia seeds and young coconut water—and now I'm about to start growing my own wheatgrass.

When I started this experiment, I had realized that I was actually killing myself with the amount and kinds of foods I was eating, but in just a short amount of time on raw, I came to understand that I could live an amazing, full life without depriving myself. Talk about gaining some mental clarity! I now have hope that life can be better than it ever was before. For the first time I truly believe that I can and will have an active, healthy, vibrant life. I've also made friends that have really helped me along this journey—real friends that I will keep for life. On August 6, I dedicated my life to living a raw food lifestyle from here on out. There's no going back now! After everything that has happened to me over the past 11 weeks, I want to do anything in my power to help promote the raw food lifestyle and community, and to support all my raw food friends.

In 11 weeks Dennis lost 64 pounds while gaining his life back. At the time of print, Dennis continues to steadily work toward his ultimate weight-loss goal and stays busy promoting the life-transforming power of the raw food diet. You can follow Dennis's progress on his healthy weight-loss journey on YouTube (see "Recommended You-Tube Channels" in the Resources section).

Resources

Recommended Raw Food and Natural Health Websites

Frank Giglio, classically trained raw food chef and personal friend, has a fantastic website that offers great recipes and many other valuable resources, including his recipe book, *Raw For All.*
FrankGiglio.com

GreenChefs bills itself as "the modern 'G' Food Network . . . featuring luscious organic and seasonal based recipes from the top Green Chefs around the world."
gliving.com/category/greenchefs

We Like It Raw is a super blog about the power of raw foods, brought to you by team lead Dhrumil Purohit and "the raw food entourage."
Welikeitraw.com

The Renegade Health Show, with hosts Kevin and Annmarie Gianni, is a fun and informative daily health show that is changing the perception of health across the world.
renegadehealth.com/blog/

Color Wheel Meals is a healthy raw food education site for the whole family, with the motto "Feed Your Kids the Color Wheel Way!" Color Wheel Meals was created by health educator and mom Samantha Gibbs.
ColorWheelMeals.com

Sunshine Boatright's website offers raw food support and education for families dealing with autism and special needs.
sunshineboatright.com

Real Food Tulsa is my regularly updated lifestyle blog. Please follow me here for all the latest information on what I'm doing at home and within the raw food world.
realfoodtulsa.com

RAW FOOD CLEANSE SUPPORT COMMUNITY ON THE WEB:
RawFoodRehab.com

RECOMMENDED YOUTUBE CHANNELS:
Anthony Anderson
http://www.youtube.com/user/Rawmodel

Dennis Clark
http://www.youtube.com/user/jdplatinum1964

Eva Gapski
http://www.youtube.com/user/LucumaPrincess

Philip McCluskey
http://www.youtube.com/user/LovingRaw

Matt Monarch & Angela Stokes Monarch
http://www.youtube.com/user/TheRawFoodWorld

Lowanna 100% Raw
   http://www.youtube.com/user/Tynx

Rawdawg Rory
   http://www.youtube.com/user/xmantidx

NATURAL BODY AND SKIN CARE PRODUCTS:

NaturalZing.com

OneLuckyDuck.com

RawEssentials.com

NATURAL CLEANING PRODUCTS FOR YOUR HOME:

Ecover.com

MethodHome.com

SeventhGeneration.com

(And of course, baking soda and vinegar)

Helpful Equipment and Gadgets for Your Raw Food Kitchen

All you really need is a good knife and a cutting board, but some of the other trinkets can be a help and make it lots of fun! I will tell you my personal preferences and a source to find each.

Knives: A good chef's knife is your most essential tool. I recommend Global (global-knife.com) or Kyocera (kyoceraadvancedceramics.com).

Cutting board: I like the products at totallybamboo.com.

Bamboo sushi mat: Makes raw vegan sushi-rolling fun and easy. You can find one of these at a restaurant supply store.

High-power blender: I use the Vita-Mix (vitamix.com).

Coffee grinder: These are good for grinding whole seeds and spices (Target, Walmart).

Dehydrator: I recommend the Excalibur (excalibur dehydrator.com).

Food processors and ice-cream makers: I recommend Cuisinart products (cuisinart.com). Bed, Bath & Beyond carries Cuisinart food processors and ice-cream makers.

Juicer: I recommend Juice Man (which you can find at Dillard's and Target), Breville (Bed, Bath & Beyond or Williams-Sonoma), Omega (omegajuicers.com) or Green Star (greenstar.com).

Mandoline: I recommend the Benriner brand. Go to the Cutlery and More website (cutleryandmore.com) and search for "Benriner."

Mason/Kerr/Ball jars: For food storage and sprouting. You can find these at most large grocery stores.

Spiral slicer: Natural Zing carries both the Saladacco and the Spirooli (naturalzing.com).

Various gadgets: Bowls, glass containers, julienne peeler, spatulas, etc. You can find many of these products at Bed, Bath & Beyond (bedbathandbeyond.com).

Raw Food Staples

RECOMMENDED ONLINE SOURCES FOR SUPPLIES:

MountainRoseHerbs.com (rose hydrosol)

NaturalZing.com

RawFoodWorld.com

PANTRY STAPLES:
Black peppercorns
Bragg Liquid Aminos
Carob and/or cacao powder
Celtic or Himalayan sea salt
Dried coconut flakes
Dried fruit and raw nuts
Nama shoyu
Raw nut butters
Spices and herbs (organic when possible)
Sun-dried tomatoes
Tahini
Vanilla extract or powder

IN YOUR REFRIGERATOR:
Bee pollen
Cold-pressed oils: hempseed, flax, olive, Udo's Choice
Kombucha
Miso, unpasteurized
Nut and seed flours
Raw olives
Unpasteurized, raw cheese

NATURAL SWEETENERS:
Agave nectar
Honey, local and raw
Maple syrup
Stevia

SEA VEGETABLES:
Dulse
Kelp
Kelp noodles

Kombu
Nori sheets
Wakame

SPECIALIZED SUPPLEMENTS AND SUPERFOODS:

Chia seeds
Digestive enzymes
Flaxseeds
Goji berries
Hemp seeds
Maca powder
Nutritional yeast
Probiotic powder
Psyllium powder

VINEGARS:

Raw apple cider vinegar
Umeboshi (plum) vinegar

References

CHAPTER 1

"Women and the Truth about Heart Health," by Connie Allen, RN, http://www.irmc.org/body.cfm?id=1398; originally published in *The Greater Lansing Business Monthly*, July 2007.

The China Study, by T. Colin Campbell (Dallas, TX: Benbella Books, 2006).

Prescription drug deaths: http://www.naturalnews.com/009278.html

"Serious adverse drug events reported to the Food and Drug Administration, 1998–2005," by T.J. Moore, M.R. Cohen, and C.D. Furberg, Archives of Internal Medicine 2007; 167:1752–1759.

http://www.findingdulcinea.com/news/health/2009/august/Americans-Taking-Alternative-Approaches-to-Health-Care.html

http://www.wellnesswithin.com/articles/pottingers%20cats.pdf

Beyond the 120 Year Diet, by Roy Walford, MD (New York: Perseus Publishing, 2000).

History of the Beverage Industry study: http://memory. loc.gov/ammem/ccmphtml/ indsthst.html

http://www.sixwise.com/newsletters/05/10/19/all-the-health-risks-of-processed-foods——in-just-a-few-quick-convenient-bites.htm

http://www.articlesbase.com/nutrition-articles/dangers-of-processed-foods-830964.html

http://articles.mercola.com/sites/articles/archive/2005/02/19/common-toxins.aspx

CHAPTER 2

http://articles.mercola.com/sites/articles/archive/2005/02/19/common-toxins.aspx

http://www.bmj.com/cgi/content/extract/328/7437/447?eaf=

http://www.hightechhealth.com/html/toxic_world.htm

Cross Currents: The Perils of Electropollution, the Promise of Electromedicine, by Robert O. Becker, MD (New York: Jeremy P. Tarcher, Inc., 1990).

http://www.bluezones.com/belong/106-feature-you-dont-have-to-be-a-nun-to-get-into-the-habit

CHAPTER 3

http://www.naturalnews.com/019957.html

http://image.examiner.com/x-12227-DC-Organic-Food-Examiner~y2009m8d11-Organics-101-What-is-the-dif-ference-between-conventional-and-organic-produce

http://www.gerson.org/g_therapy/default.asp

http://jn.nutrition.org/cgi/content/abstract/34/5/507

The pH Miracle: Balance Your Diet, Reclaim Your Health, by Robert O. Young and Shelley Redford Young (New York: Warner Books, 2002).

http://www.mayoclinic.com/health/water/NU00283/ NSECTIONGROUP=2

http://www.articlesbase.com/alternative-medicine-articles/why-acidalkaline-body-balance-is-a-must-497694.html

http://juicefeasting.com/92Days/Days1120/Day17Bee PollenandBVitamins/tabid/99/Default.aspx

http://www.juicefeasting.com/JuiceFeastingSpectrum Intro/SupplementsandSuperfoods/tabid/182/ Default.aspx

http://www.hippocratesinst.org/Wheatgrass.aspx

CHAPTER 5

Recipe contributors:
Robin Abbott
Wendy Agee
Delaney Berrini
Katie Boydston
Susan Bradbury
Stacey Bradford
Andrea Crossman
Janine Gibbons
Frank Giglio
Pamela Girouard
Kimberly Graham
Amie Sue Oldfather
Heather Stiltz

CHAPTER 6

http://guineapiglets.ning.com/forum/topics/saturdays-thread

http://articles.mercola.com/sites/articles/archive/2005/02/19/common-toxins.aspx

CHAPTER 7

Return to the Sacred, by Jonathan Ellerby, PhD (Carlsbad, CA, Hay House, Inc., 2009).

Handbook of Religion and Health, by Koenig, McCollough and Larson (New York, Oxford University Press, 2001).

The Blue Zones, by Dan Buettner (Des Moines, IA, National Geographic Publishing, 2008).

"Beneficial Effects of Sun Exposure on Cancer Mortality," by Gordon Ainsleigh (Netherlands, American Journal of Preventive Medicine, 1993).

http://topten.org/public/BN/BN183.html

http://www.holisticonline.com/Yoga/hol_yoga_breathing_Importance.htm

http://www.mayoclinic.com/health/walking/HQ01612

http://www.healthandyoga.com/html/yoga/Benefits.html

http://www.healingdaily.com/exercise/rebounding-for-detoxification-and-health.htm

http://www.jashbotanicals.com/articles/skin_brushing.html

http://www.basabody.com/health-benefits-of-coconut-oil.html

References

http://www.whatreallyworks.co.uk/start/articles.asp?
   article_ID=451

http://longevity.about.com/od/lifelongenergy/tp/
   healthy_sleep.htm

http://www.biohealthinfo.com/html/resources/
   4pillars/sleep.html#top

http://www.mind-and-body-yoga.com/sleep-benefits.
   html

http://www.totalhealthlife.com/about.html

http://www.medicinenet.com/script/main/art.asp?
   articlekey=50874

http://www.faithmag.com/faithmag/column2.asp?
   ArticleID=931

Recipe Index

A

Almond Cacao Truffles, 99–100
Andrea's Awesome E.A.T.
    Sandwich, 132–33
Anemia Buster, 104–105
Apple Rosemary Infusion, 116
Asian Cucumber Salad, 73–74

B

Balancing Broth, 76–77
Basic Black, 108
Beggin' Strips, 89
Berries Unite, 53–54
Berry Bliss, 56–57
The Best Guacamole, 83–84
Black Beans & Rice, 131
Blended Bruschetta, 82–83
Blood Orange Raw Mojito, 113
Blue Moon, 110
Blueberry Hemp-Nut Shake, 59
Bradbury's Tropical Smoothie, 110

Breakfasts, 118–21
Butternut Sage Spaghetti, 93–94

C

Cacao Banana, 112
Cacao Maca Ice Cream—for Raw
    Food Superheroes!, 140
Cashew Cheese, 84
The Charmer and the Kale, 57
Cheesy Broccoli & Cauliflower,
    128–29
Chia Coconut Custard Shake, 56
Chia Seed Ice Cream, 100
Chilled Cucumber Soup, 80
Chocotini, 115
Cilantro Lime Dressing, 65
Citrus Basil Infusion, 62–63
Citrus Blast, 103–104
Clean Sweep, 105
Clear & Calm, 104
Cocktails, 60–62, 112–16
Corn Tortilla Chips, 89–90

Cream of Asparagus Soup, 124
Creamy Avocado Soup, 77
Creamy Macadamia Dressing,
    65–66

D

Decadent Chocomole, 138
Delaney's Soft-serve Banana Ice
    Cream, 100–101
Desserts, 99–102, 136–40
Digestive Healer, 111
Dreamsicle Shake, 110
Dressings, 116–18
Dressings, 65–68

E

Easy Raw Hummus, 85–86
Ecstatic Elixirs, 62–65
Egg-free "Egg Nog" Smoothie, 111
Entrées, 129–36
Entrées, 90–99
Exotic Endurance, 57

F

Fiesta Salad, 68–69
French Dressing, 66–67
Fresh Corn & Tomato Salad, 70–71
Fruit 'n' Fiber, 58
Fuzzy Navel, 114

G

Garden Variety, 47
Garden Wraps, 96
Garden-Fresh Chilled Summer
    Salad, 71
Gentle Liver-Cleanse Smoothie,
    55–56
Get Lucky Green Juice, 48
Get Your Green On, 108

Ginger-Peach Bellini, 61
Goji High, 58
Good Vibrations Salad, 69
Gracious Grains with Voluptuous
    Veggies, 135
Green Beauty, 48–49
Green Curry, 81
Green Drink, 46–47
Green Gringo, 52–53
Green Mechanic, 52
The Green Smoothie, 55

H

Healthy Hound, 61–62
Herb-ocado, 78
Hipped-Up Sweet Potato Cashew
    Casserole, 132
Homemade Chili-in-the-Raw,
    130–31
Honey Lime Vinaigrette, 117–18
Honey Mustard Dressing, 67

I

I Can See Now, 106
Indian Curry Silk, 123
Island Flush, 54

J

Janine Gibbons' Jicama Lime
    Salad, 75
Janine's Pineapple Thai Salad,
    72–73
Juices, 46–54, 103–107
Juicy Pink, 103

K

Katie's Blueberry Crumble, 120
Katie's Coconut Chia Fruit
    Smoothie, 59

Killer Summer Celery Soup, 81–82
Kumquat Caipiroska, 114

L

Lemon Rescue, 57–58
Lemony Licorice, 64–65
Liquid Gazpacho, 78–89
Liquid Salad, 48
Liquid Sunshine, 106
Loaded Cucumbers, 95

M

Manna Bread Layered Breakfast
    Toast, 120–21
Marinated Asparagus, 71–72
Marinated Broccoli, 75
Market Fresh Tomato Soup, 77
Marvelous Marinated Bean Salad,
    128
Melon Kiwi-tini, 112–13
Minestrone, 124
Mint Julep, 113
The Mother Sauce, 116–17
Mushroom Alfredo Linguine,
    92–93
My Daily Green, 47
My Green Goddess, 51

N

Nectar of the Mexican Goddesses,
    122–23

O

Ocean Goddess Heartland Mud
    "Pie," 101
One Hot Ruby, 54
Orange Spinach Salad with
    Orange Tahini Dressing, 69–70
Orange-ango, 108

P

Pamela's Key Lime Pie, 137
Pamela's Original Apple-Pie
    Salad, 138–39
Pasta with Leeks, Radicchio,
    Walnut Pesto & Parmesan,
    129–30
Peaches & Crème, 111–12
Penni-colada, 109
Penni's Patio Salad, 83
Penni's Pesto, 84–85
Penni's Picnic Potato Salad,
    126–27
Pesto Italiano, 125
Pico de Gallo, 49–50
Pineapple-Jalapeño Coleslaw, 73
Portobello Burgers by Amie Sue,
    133–34
Portobello Steaks with Wilted
    Spinach Salad, 98–99
Protein Purifier, 107
Pure Vitality, 105
Purple Passion, 53

Q

Quinoa Tabbouleh with
    Pistachios, 125–26

R

Raspberry Love, 58
Raw Ketchup, 117
Raw Marinated Vegetable Salad,
    74
Raw Morning Power Bars, 119
Raw Mustard, 67
Raw Zucchini Pasta with Fresh
    Marinara, 91–92
Razzle Dazzle, 60–61
"Roasted" Red Bell Pepper
    Hummus, 86–87
Robin Abbott's Tomato Stacks, 97

Rosie Rooibos, 64
Ruby's Raw Cherry Granola, 118–19
Ruby's Smokin' Hot Tomato Soup, 122
The Rubyvroom, 62

S

Salads, 68–75, 125–29
Sassy Bunny, 107
Sauces, 65–68, 116–18
Seasonal Fruit Crisp, 136–37
Shakes, 55–59, 107–12
Side dishes, 83–90, 125–29
Simple Pleasure, 104
Simple Stuffed Mushrooms, 90–91
The Smart Cocktail, 60
Smoothies, 55–59, 107–12
Snacks, 83–90, 125–29
Soups, 76–83, 121-24
Spiced (Not Spiked) Holiday Punch, 115–16
Spicy Green Tomato, 50–51
Spring Green Goodness, 49
Spring Rolls with Peanut Sauce, 95–96
Sprouted Lentils with Greens and Pistachio Pesto, 92
Stacey Bradford's Nacho Dip, 87
Stacey's Lemon Tahini Dressing or Dip, 67–68
Stone Temple Purifier, 51–52
Strawberry Cloud, 121–22
Stuffed Baked Potato Supper, 135–36
Stuffed Bell Peppers, 94
Sun & Sea Pâté, 85
Sun-dried Tomato & Jalapeño Hummus, 86
Supermodel Blend, 108–109

Susan's Delicious Raw Carrot Cake, 101–102
Susan's Kale Chips 2.0, 88–89
Susan's Onion Bread, 90
Susan's Scrumptious Living Chocolate Cheesecake, 139–40
Sweet & Spicy Kale Chips, 88
Sweet Basil, 106–107

T

Tabbouleh in a Bowl, 79
Taco Salad Platter, 97
Tahini Dressing 2.0, 68
Tangy Green Tease, 103
Thai Green Transfusion, 50
Thai Salad Dressing, 66
Thai Soup, 80–81
"Thousand Island," 66
Tomatillo Salsa Verde, 79

V

Veggie Chowder, 82
Virgin Mary, 60–61

W

Warrior Blend, 109
WendiLou's Berries & Cream, 99
White Bean Dip, 126
Wild Greek Salad, 70
Wild Rice Salad, 127–28
Wild Thing, 55

Y

Yerba Latte, 63–64

Other Books from Ulysses Press

THE GREEN SMOOTHIES DIET: THE NATURAL PROGRAM FOR
EXTRAORDINARY HEALTH
Robyn Openshaw, $14.95
Offers a program complete with recipes for transforming
one's health by drinking green smoothies. While fruit
smoothies are fine, this book explains why smoothies
made from both fruit and greens, the ultimate superfoods,
can improve all aspects of one's health and add years to
one's life.

THE COMPLETE MASTER CLEANSE: A STEP-BY-STEP GUIDE
TO MAXIMIZING THE BENEFITS OF THE LEMONADE DIET
Tom Woloshyn, $13.95
Fasting while drinking a blend of clear spring water,
cayenne pepper and citrus juice has proven to be a safe,
simple and yet powerful way to cleanse the body of toxins. This book goes beyond basic information by guiding
readers step by step through the entire cleansing process.

SUGAR-FREE GLUTEN-FREE BAKING AND DESSERTS:
RECIPES FOR HEALTHY AND DELICIOUS COOKIES, CAKES,
MUFFINS, SCONES, PIES, PUDDINGS, BREADS AND PIZZAS
Kelly Keough, $14.95
Shows readers how to bring taboo treats back to the baking sheet with savory recipes that swap wheat for whole-
some alternatives like quinoa, arrowroot and tapioca
starch, and trade in sugar for natural sweeteners like
agave, yacon and stevia.

THE GI MEDITERRANEAN DIET: THE GLYCEMIC INDEX-
BASED LIFE-SAVING DIET OF THE GREEKS
Dr. Fedon Alexander Lindberg, $14.95
Mediterranean cuisine and GI dieting are a proven match
made in culinary heaven. This book shows readers how

the Old World's most celebrated foods can keep you lean, young and living a longer and healthier life.

THE JUICE FASTING BIBLE: DISCOVER THE POWER OF AN ALL-JUICE DIET TO RESTORE GOOD HEALTH, LOSE WEIGHT AND INCREASE VITALITY
Dr. Sandra Cabot, $12.95
Offering a series of quick and easy juice fasts, this book provides a reader-friendly approach to an increasingly popular alternative health practice.

RAW JUICING: THE HEALTHY, EASY AND DELICIOUS WAY TO GAIN THE BENEFITS OF THE RAW FOOD LIFESTYLE
Leslie Kenton, $12.95
As the health benefits of eating uncooked food becomes widely acknowledge, more people are looking for ways to "go raw." This book's raw-juice plan and great-tasting recipes offers the easiest way to "go raw" for a meal: make a super-healthy, delicious raw juice drink.

THE PH BALANCE DIET: RESTORE YOUR ACID-ALKALINE LEVELS TO ELIMINATE TOXINS AND LOSE WEIGHT
Bharti Vyas & Suzanne Le Quesne, $12.95
Tells how to pH-test one's body, correct imbalances, and eliminate toxic overload by following a dietary way of life that works. An easy-to-follow section with over 40 recipes is included to help guide readers through the plan.

To order these books call 800-377-2542 or 510-601-8301, fax 510-601-8307, e-mail ulysses@ulyssespress.com, or write to Ulysses Press, P.O. Box 3440, Berkeley, CA 94703. All retail orders are shipped free of charge. California residents must include sales tax. Allow two to three weeks for delivery.

About the Author

Penni Shelton has a powerful story of healing from IBS, her lifelong, debilitating condition, through embracing a diet rich in raw and living foods. Her restoration story began in 2004 and was first published in Carol Alt's book *The Raw 50*. Penni facilitates raw food education both locally and internationally, focusing her passion on creating a sense of community and support within health-conscious circles. She is an avid raw food and lifestyle writer at the website RealFoodTulsa.com, has been interviewed by and written for a variety of natural health publications and websites, and has published an e-book, *Raw for the Holidays*. She currently stays busy running her international-community website RawFoodRehab.com. Penni lives in Tulsa, Oklahoma, with her husband and two children.